Steve writes like he speaks and speaks like he lives, taking the reader on a ride through his life experiences and subsequent lessons. This is more of a confession than a sermon; more a voyage of discovery than a discourse. Steve Willis is to be commended for addressing this national issue in a holistic fashion, and offering no-nonsense directions anyone can follow.

Allan Thompson, Ph.D.
Director, Great Commission Center
East Texas Baptist University
Marshall, Texas

STEVE WILLIS

WINNING THE FOOD FIGHT

WITH KEN WALKER

Victory in the Physical and Spiritual Battle for
Good Food and a Healthy Lifestyle

Regal

From Gospel Light
Ventura, California, U.S.A.

Published by Regal
From Gospel Light
Ventura, California, U.S.A.
www.regalbooks.com
Printed in the U.S.A.

Willis, Steve.
Winning the food fight : victory in the physical and spiritual battle for good food
and a healthy lifestyle / Steve Willis with Ken Walker.
p. cm.
ISBN 978-0-8307-6122-7 (hard cover)
1. Food—Religious aspects—Christianity. 2. Health—Religious aspects—Christianity.
3. Weight loss—Religious aspects—Christianity. I. Walker, Ken, 1957- II. Title.
BR115.N87W56 2011
248.4—dc23
2011037308

Rights for publishing this book outside the U.S.A. or in non-English languages are administered
by Gospel Light Worldwide, an international not-for-profit ministry. For additional information,
please visit www.glww.org, email info@glww.org, or write to Gospel Light Worldwide,
1957 Eastman Avenue, Ventura, CA 93003, U.S.A.

To order copies of this book and other Regal products in bulk quantities,
please contact us at 1-800-446-7735.

To my wife, Deanna,
who cared about our children's health
long before I "got it."

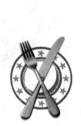

Contents

Foreword by Jamie Oliver 9

Preface 11

Acknowledgments 13

Round 1   The Call 15

Round 2   Weighed Down 29

Round 3   Does God Really Care? 43

Round 4   A Biblical Plan for Change 61

Round 5   The Man in the Mirror 75

Round 6   There's No Place Like Home 89

Round 7   Our Church Isn't Growing (And We're Happy About It)............107

Round 8   It's Taking a Village..123

Round 9   Back to School 139

Round 10   The Politics of Food...153

Round 11   Life in the Fast(ing) Lane....................................173

Round 12   It's Not Business; It's Personal 191

Recipes by Jamie Oliver 207

Resources 215

Endnotes 219

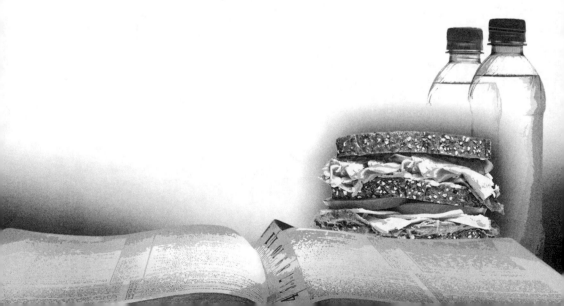

Foreword

By Jamie Oliver

Pastor Steve and I share a common goal: He wants to inspire his community to be healthier and have a better relationship with food, and I want to inspire people around the world to question what they are eating and consider what their dietary choices are doing to their health.

The fact is that diet-related disease is killing Pastor Steve's community. Because of that, he's put this brilliant book together. It's a patchwork quilt made up of many different stories from his community as well as his personal experiences of the Food Revolution—a process that we've only just begun.

We have both faced the day-to-day reality of the devastation caused by the obesity epidemic in the United Kingdom and the United States. Diet-related disease is the biggest killer in America and the costliest to the American health care system. One in three Americans is overweight or obese, and we now know that this will be the first generation where children are expected to live shorter lives than their parents. We live in a time when five-year-olds are having their teeth removed because of gum disease caused by a reliance on soda pop as their only source of hydration.

It's time to change the way we treat ourselves, the way we nourish our families and the way we buy food. We need to think about where that food comes from, how it's made, what impact that has on the world around us, and the future choices of our children's children. We need to reconnect with real food and start placing value on basic cooking skills so that people are properly equipped to feed themselves.

I spent the early part of 2011 carrying on the work of the Food Revolution in Los Angeles, and what I experienced there made me even prouder of the community in Huntington, West Virginia, and the Tri-state area where we first began our campaign. The community at large has carried on with the work we started and has achieved more than we ever imagined. Huntington has become a symbol of what *is* possible. I humbly salute them.

During a particularly rough patch, Pastor Steve advised me to stay strong and stick to my beliefs. Then he said something I've never forgotten: "Nobody changes until the pain of staying the same becomes greater than the pain of change itself." Never a truer word has been spoken. Just because some things are hard, slow and painful doesn't mean that you should stop doing what you know in your heart is right. The things that inspire me have nothing to do with the future; they are little bits of good information from the past—the stuff your great-grandmother would have known, like how something you've cooked yourself will taste 100 times better than something that comes out of a box or on a fast-food tray.

So, lovely people, please enjoy this book that has been passionately put together by our main man, the one and only Pastor Steve. I hope it will inspire you to do things differently, and maybe even engage as a member of the community by acting as a Food Revolutionary yourself. I'm proud to be able to support Pastor Steve and his book. He speaks with the voice of reason, and he talks to his community not only as a pastor but also as a friend.

Big love,
Jamie

Preface

This book is not just for those who need to lose weight, although reading it will help. Nor is it solely for mothers who want to do what is best for their children, although reading it should help there too. Even though I am a pastor, I did not write this book just for people of faith. Why? Because the food fight confronting our nation affects people of every race, gender, personal belief and socio-economic level. You name it, it concerns us all.

Winning the Food Fight is intended for anyone who cares about the health of their family, the wellbeing of their community, and the future of our nation. You may consider that an exaggeration. After you read this book, however, I think you will agree that the battle being waged over food is a fight that we must win—sooner rather than later.

There are few things that are as tantalizing, satisfying and enjoyable as a delicious meal. However, like any other substance, pastime or avocation, too much of a good thing can ruin us. From the beginning of human history, we have struggled to say no to the wrong things. Like our ancestors Adam and Eve, we struggle to walk away from that which is "pleasing to the eye" (Gen. 3:6). Because of this, the food God created to sustain and strengthen us has been transformed into something that now leads millions to an early grave. That which He created to give life inflicts pain instead.

To put it bluntly, I wrote *Winning the Food Fight* because I am tired of watching people die before their time. I am tired of seeing too many young families weighed down by the mental, spiritual, emotional and physical burdens of poor eating habits. I am tired of seeing children fail to reach their potential because they have been given too much junk food and not enough nutrition. As a pastor, I am tired of seeing the lives of people I love get cut short or who barely exist during their golden years because they lack the education, discipline or resources they need to make wise dietary choices.

We *can* do better. We *must* do better. As you read this book, I pray that your heart will break as you consider truths about a dietary system whose deadly impact has devastated individuals and families. The news isn't all bad, however. You will also see numerous stories about people who took charge of their food choices and today are doing better. Much better. You will also hear how people living in what had been labeled the "unhealthiest city in America" are changing, and you will learn how your community can take similar steps.

You are about to wade into the ring. Brace yourself. In this society, you will hear a chorus of discouraging words from people who say you can't win this fight, you shouldn't care about it, and you *deserve* all those foods that are harmful to your health. Don't listen to them. Join me on a journey that will show you how you can overcome the foe that wants to weigh you down and send you to an early grave.

Acknowledgments

This book would not have been possible apart from the support of . . .

My wife, Deanna, and our three children, Titus, Johnna and Lucas. Sorry for all the times you had to maintain silence in the house so I could keep writing.

The shepherds and congregation of First Baptist Kenova. There would be no story here if you hadn't jumped on board.

My mother and father. The road has been rocky at best, but your wagon rolls on. Keep on keeping on.

The administrators of the Bowen Trust and the Baptist churches of West Virginia. You funded nearly all of my higher education. May your investment continue to reap great rewards.

Jamie Oliver, his staff and the producers of ABC's *Food Revolution*. You came in to make a positive difference and to tell a story that had to be broadcasted to our nation. Just because some people don't get it, do not be deterred. The cause is just.

The people of Huntington, West Virginia. The deck is stacked against us, but still we persevere. We can win the food fight.

My right-hand man in this project, Ken Walker, who used his writing talents to assemble many of this book's real-life stories that will enlighten and inspire you. Without his crafty pen and interviewing skills, this story would not have been told in a way it deserves.

The grace of the good Lord in heaven. Whatever we eat or drink, may it be to His glory.

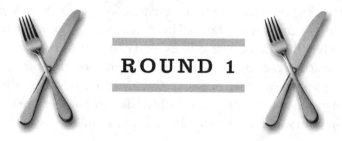

ROUND 1

The Call

Mondays get a bad rap. People typically grumble about the first day of the workweek, reflecting their yearning for more time to kick back, relax and forget the world's cares. The naysayers overlook the fact that Mondays offer all kinds of possibilities. You can resume productive activity, renew relationships in the marketplace, and move forward in meaningful occupations or other pursuits. For Huntington, West Virginia, a divinely inspired telephone call one Monday in the summer of 2009 changed the course of our history. That call got us up off the mat and into the fight.

Although I am involved in this story, I am just a bit player in a drama that reaches from coast to coast, involving every town, city, county and state in America—a nation that is slowly committing suicide. We are not killing ourselves with drugs, alcohol or guns, although each of those plays a sad role in our social deterioration. The elephant in the room—the always-present beast that most everyone knows is there but no one wants to openly acknowledge—is fat. Whether in the form of butter dripping from yeast rolls, juice oozing from a slab of prime rib, double-cheese pizzas, or sugary-sweet cakes piled high with icing and topped off with softball-sized dollops of ice cream, too much fat is a killer. Overindulging in calorie-rich, processed foods inflicts worse damage than most terrorists can conceive. America is in a food fight, and right now we are losing. Until we started to change our ways, Huntington was faring as poorly as anyone in this battle.

The toll I witnessed in our church shook me to the core. Simply persuading church leaders to let me address the problem in the summer of 2008 took considerable discussion, explanation and prayer. If there's one thing Americans do not appreciate, it is someone pointing out the damage caused by gluttonous habits. Nearly a year after we formed an initiative to help those who were severely overweight, we realized we needed help. Some folks were struggling to shed more than a few pounds. Ironically, many had hit the exercise trail like Olympic athletes. However, they hadn't adjusted their eating routines, and it was showing.

After our first "Big Losers" groups (we originally called them "Biggest Loser" groups, but changed the name because of trademark concerns) ended in late spring of 2009, I didn't know what to say or how to offer further help. I discussed my frustrations with my wife, Dee, who pointed out that she wasn't a nutrition expert either. Finally, one Sunday I prayed, "Lord, we need help. We need somebody to come and teach us nutrition. It's going to cost a lot, and we don't have the money to pay someone for that. So we're looking to You."

The next day, my assistant buzzed my office: "Pastor Willis, there's a man named Jason Skweres on line two. He says he's with ABC Television."

Wonder what he wants? I thought. After Jason introduced himself and explained he was with GCM Productions, a company based in Los Angeles, he asked if I knew Jamie Oliver. I hesitated. The name was unfamiliar to me.

"Have you ever heard of *The Naked Chef*?"

That rang a bell.

"I'm pretty sure I've heard of that show," I replied. "My wife watches the Cooking Channel. I imagine he's been on there."

"We heard about what you're doing there," Jason said, referring to media coverage of our weight-loss effort. The frequency of the stories about our church's health kick had increased exponentially after the Centers for Disease Control (CDC) issued a report pinpointing our area as the unhealthiest in the nation. One local story even wound up on network television. Apparently, we were one of the first groups or organizations in our area to attempt to address the problem.

"We work for Jamie," Jason continued, explaining that his boss was the executive producer. "He read about the CDC report that showed your area was the worst in the United States for obesity problems. He wants to come to Huntington and teach people about nutrition. He hopes to focus on helping cooks in the school lunch program prepare healthier meals and film a mini-series about it. It would be something like the one he did in 2005 about the junk food served in Britain's school lunch program. We could use a local contact to introduce us to people around town, and we hope you'll get some benefits from learning about healthy cooking."

"When are you coming?" I asked.

"In two days."

Talk about a quick answer to prayer! Jamie didn't come to film the bulk of his first *Food Revolution* mini-series for six more weeks, but in the meantime the crew had plenty of groundwork to do. They needed to explain their concept to school officials, political and community leaders, and news media. After meeting with Jason and several other producers, I felt confident that they were here to help—not to poke fun or expand the stereotypical image of Appalachians as poor, backward hillbillies. Believe me, that has been done too many times. Having grown up about 60 miles east of Huntington, I've heard more jokes and misconceptions than I care to remember. I can tell when someone wants to take potshots at us. These guys didn't.

We're Number One!

The CDC report that lured Jamie Oliver to Huntington still makes me shudder.

Local purists protested that the city itself wasn't labeled the nation's fattest; it was really a five-county area spread over three states. True, but everyone here knows that residents of West Virginia, Ohio and Kentucky living along the Ohio River freely interact, work and travel among the three states. With Huntington at the center of this five-county area, that distinction was barely worth noting. The fact was that our city and its nearest neighbors were suffering from the nation's highest rates of obesity and numerous resulting illnesses. My personal experience bore out those statistics. People were dying—and many were members of my church.

Lots of places boast about being first in athletics, academics, job creation, housing sales or retail profits. Reign at the top of one of those lists and a sense of pride fills the air. Because success breeds success, being first in one category often leads to greatness in another. Unfortunately, the same can be said of negative environments. Our area was leading the nation in the types of statistics where you *don't* want to be first. When it comes to poor health, the old "We're #1!" chant doesn't exactly rev up the fan base.

According to the CDC, we were *first* in the nation in the percentage of adults who did not exercise (31 percent), *first* in the prevalence of heart disease (22 percent), and *first* in the percentage of people who had diabetes (13 percent). Nearly half of those over age 65 did not have any of their natural teeth left (first place in that category too)! We were *first* (as in *worst*) in high blood pressure, circulation problems, kidney disease, vision problems and sleeping disorders. Did I mention that we were *first* in rates of depression? While other cities may have come close to our percentages in some categories, no one else touched the whopping 46 percent of adults who were obese.[1]

Think about that. Nearly one out of every two adults in our area was obese—not just overweight, but obese. An "obese" person is someone with a body mass index (BMI) of at least 30. The chart on page 21 demonstrates how to calculate BMI using height and weight, with a healthy BMI being less than 25. That means a man who is 5 feet, 10 inches tall needs to weigh 173 pounds or less to meet this standard. Anyone of that height who weighs 209 or above fits the definition of obesity. Right now, many are gasping, "You've got to be kidding!" That is because we are so used to overweight people that many folks consider healthy people to be too skinny—possibly even wondering if they suffer from a strange disease or eating disorder.

By and large (pun intended), America as a whole is not far behind the Huntington area in most categories. We may be the worst, but we are encamped within the most obese region (the Southeast) in the most obese nation in the world. In 2010, an expert panel conducting research for the United States Department of Agriculture (USDA) asserted that obesity posed the single greatest threat to public health in this century. Former Surgeon General Richard Carmona once stated it more strongly: "Obesity is the terror within," he said during a lecture at the University of South Carolina. "Unless we do something about it, the magnitude of the dilemma will dwarf 9-11 or any other terrorist attempt."[2]

In a separate interview, Dr. Carmona stated, "Obesity is absolutely at the core of the chronic disease crisis. When we look at the relationship of obesity to other diseases that plague society today (such as asthma, cancer, cardiovascular disease, and diabetes) obesity increases the incidence of each of them, and can even accelerate some of them. Losing weight is not about trying to emulate models in fashion magazines, it's about being healthy. If we could only address one major public health issue as a nation, I would focus on the obesity crisis. Weight loss could have the greatest impact in decreasing the chronic disease burden in America."[3]

Dr. Carmona may sound like an alarmist, but ring the bell he should. The CDC predicts that one out of three children born in America in the year 2000 will develop Type II diabetes.[4] We're not talking about the common cold; one in three Americans will be in the high-risk category for heart attacks, strokes, blindness, nerve damage and amputations. In addition, the American Cancer Society warns that up to 60 percent of cancers are related to lifestyle choices, such as how well we eat and whether or not we get adequate exercise.[5] The evidence keeps piling up. Whether it is cancer of the breast, colon, uterus, esophagus or kidney, obesity increases our likelihood of dying from these diseases.

Ironically, even though we all know that overeating is bad for us and too much weight may kill us, each year we spend increasing amounts of money eating out. This habit even spills over to our pets. One in four American dogs and cats is now obese.[6] I sometimes wonder when animal rights activists will start picketing fast-food restaurants and all-you-can-eat buffets to call more attention to this sad state of helpless pets (after all, they don't feed themselves). Meanwhile, children in Africa are dying for lack of food and other necessary resources. Imagine trying to explain that one on judgment day!

Dr. David Kessler served as Commissioner of the U.S. Food and Drug Administration under Presidents George H. W. Bush and Bill Clinton. A pediatrician, Dr. Kessler has also served as the dean of the medical schools at Yale University and the University of California, San Francisco. He is an alumnus of Amherst College, the University of Chicago Law School, and Harvard Medical School. Given his résumé, perhaps we should listen to what he has to say about our nation's love affair with food: "When we talk about the complexity of American foods, we aren't referring to the kind of complexity traditionally associated with fine cuisine or regional or ethnic cooking. The American concept of complexity is built on layering and loading [with sugars, fats and salt], rather than an intricate and subtle use of quality ingredients."[7] In *The End of Overeating*, Kessler suggests that major changes need to take place in American food systems—or else our nation is heading for a health care disaster. I have seen what disaster looks like in Huntington—and as I mentioned earlier, though we might be the worst in the country, most states are statistically just a few years behind.

We are in quite a conundrum. While we overeat, the bulk of the foods we consume do not give us the nutrients we need. We have tons of choices at our fingertips, but instead of improving our health, our food is destroying us. What *are* we going to do? What *can* we do? In the face of such a monumental problem, any one individual's attempt to address it may seem futile. I used to feel the same way. When I raised the issue in our church, I never dreamed that one day my sermon would be broadcast nationwide. Even as I prepared the outline, I asked myself, *What can one person do in the face of such a staggering situation?* At that moment, I had to gather my resolve and determine to do what I could and leave the rest in God's hands.

Body Mass Index Table

	Normal						Overweight					Obese										Extreme Obesity														
BMI	19	20	21	22	23	24	25	26	27	28	29	30	31	32	33	34	35	36	37	38	39	40	41	42	43	44	45	46	47	48	49	50	51	52	53	54
Height (inches)												Body Weight (pounds)																								
58	91	96	100	105	110	115	119	124	129	134	138	143	148	153	158	162	167	172	177	181	186	191	196	201	205	210	215	220	224	229	234	239	244	248	253	258
59	94	99	104	109	114	119	124	128	133	138	143	148	153	158	163	168	173	178	183	188	193	198	203	208	212	217	222	227	232	237	242	247	252	257	262	267
60	97	102	107	112	118	123	128	133	138	143	148	153	158	163	168	174	179	184	189	194	199	204	209	215	220	225	230	235	240	245	250	255	261	266	271	276
61	100	106	111	116	122	127	132	137	143	148	153	158	164	169	174	180	185	190	195	201	206	211	217	222	227	232	238	243	248	254	259	264	269	275	280	285
62	104	109	115	120	126	131	136	142	147	153	158	164	169	175	180	186	191	196	202	207	213	218	224	229	235	240	246	251	256	262	267	273	278	284	289	295
63	107	113	118	124	130	135	141	146	152	158	163	169	175	180	186	191	197	203	208	214	220	225	231	237	242	248	254	259	265	270	278	282	287	293	299	304
64	110	116	122	128	134	140	145	151	157	163	169	174	180	186	192	197	204	209	215	221	227	232	238	244	250	256	262	267	273	279	285	291	296	302	308	314
65	114	120	126	132	138	144	150	156	162	168	174	180	186	192	198	204	210	216	222	228	234	240	246	252	258	264	270	276	282	288	294	300	306	312	318	324
66	118	124	130	136	142	148	155	161	167	173	179	186	192	198	204	210	216	223	229	235	241	247	253	260	266	272	278	284	291	297	303	309	315	322	328	334
67	121	127	134	140	146	153	159	166	172	178	185	191	198	204	211	217	223	230	236	242	249	255	261	268	274	280	287	293	299	306	312	319	325	331	338	344
68	125	131	138	144	151	158	164	171	177	184	190	197	203	210	216	223	230	236	243	249	256	262	269	276	282	289	295	302	308	315	322	328	335	341	348	354
69	128	135	142	149	155	162	169	176	182	189	196	203	209	216	223	230	236	243	250	257	263	270	277	284	291	297	304	311	318	324	331	338	345	351	358	365
70	132	139	146	153	160	167	174	181	188	195	202	209	216	222	229	236	243	250	257	264	271	278	285	292	299	306	313	320	327	334	341	348	355	362	369	376
71	136	143	150	157	165	172	179	186	193	200	208	215	222	229	236	243	250	257	265	272	279	286	293	301	308	315	322	329	338	343	351	358	365	372	379	386
72	140	147	154	162	169	177	184	191	199	206	213	221	228	235	242	250	258	265	272	279	287	294	302	309	316	324	331	338	346	353	361	368	375	383	390	397
73	144	151	159	166	174	182	189	197	204	212	219	227	235	242	250	257	265	272	280	288	295	302	310	318	325	333	340	348	355	363	371	378	386	393	401	408
74	148	155	163	171	179	186	194	202	210	218	225	233	241	249	256	264	272	280	287	295	303	311	319	326	334	342	350	358	365	373	381	389	396	404	412	420
75	152	160	168	176	184	192	200	208	216	224	232	240	248	256	264	272	279	287	295	303	311	319	327	335	343	351	359	367	375	383	391	399	407	415	423	431
76	156	164	172	180	189	197	205	213	221	230	238	246	254	263	271	279	287	295	304	312	320	328	336	344	353	361	369	377	385	394	402	410	418	426	435	443

Source: Adapted from *Clinical Guidelines on the Identification, Evaluation, and Treatment of Overweight and Obesity in Adults: The Evidence Report*

After all, if history has taught us anything, it is this: If a few passionate individuals invest their faith and energy in a cause greater than self, then the One who is greater than any human being can use those individuals to bring about real change—a revolution. History is full of revolutions that have changed the destinies of peoples and nations. I saw no reason why the same could not happen here and now. So as I led our church to participate in *Jamie Oliver's Food Revolution*, I appreciated the deep spiritual significance of the program's title.

Overcoming Suspicion

Given our negative health statistics, you might expect that someone who wanted to help us turn things around would be welcomed cordially. Not so. Suspicion, misgivings and sometimes outright hostility greeted Jamie's producers as they circulated around the Tri-state area. Many people were reluctant to accept the fact that we were in such bad condition. The last thing they wanted was more negative attention brought to our doorstep.

At first, no political leaders would endorse such a show, fearing it might portray the area in a bad light. Few others were willing to dip their toes in the water. Overall, I'd characterize the attitude as: *If there's a problem here, we can fix it ourselves.* I managed to convince a few community leaders that the producers were decent folks and didn't want to harm us, but it took awhile for many residents to warm up to the idea.

The disc jockey with the area's most popular radio station spent the first few episodes carping at Jamie, symbolizing those who greeted the outsiders with clenched fists. The negative reactions, blunt disbelief, and "Who are you to come in here and tell us anything?" attitude weren't acts for the cameras. Neither was the critical reception Jamie received at the elementary school cafeteria featured in the early episodes. (I couldn't get too upset with the skeptics. Changing the way we eat costs money, arouses controversy and stirs the pot, so to speak. Some resistance was probably inevitable—and even though such friction can be quite uncomfortable, it often sparks progress.)

Still, if you think that dealing with this kind of reception to a well-intentioned effort is easy, it is only because you haven't faced such opposition. More than once, Jamie asked if he could take a break to blow off steam or confide in me about the pressures he was facing. Not only did he have to wade through emotionally laden opposition, but also his series would air before a national audience. Without some breakthroughs, the effort could collapse. Besides there being millions of dollars on the line and network executives expecting a first-class production, Jamie had staked his reputation on this show. Tackling the project also kept him away from his wife and three children (they have since had a fourth) for several weeks. As a father of three who has spent considerable time away from home on mission trips and ministry travel, I understood his angst.

Jamie Oliver is essentially the same person in real life as he is on TV, although he turns up the personality when the cameras roll. That isn't phony; I do the same thing when I step into the pulpit. When you're passionate about something, you get excited when you have an opportunity to tell others about it. Besides, if I don't communicate passion for the topic on which I'm preaching, few listeners are going to care what I say. It's the same way for Jamie. If he isn't witty, charming, interesting and vivacious when filming material, viewers will reach for the remote control a few minutes into his program. Fortunately, despite early obstacles, that didn't happen with our show in Huntington. The series drew anywhere from 3.91 million to 7.51 million viewers during its six-week run in the spring of 2010, peaking during the second round of the NCAA basketball tournament. The program impressed the industry too, capturing that year's Emmy Award for "Outstanding Reality TV Program."

Jamie featured a part of my obesity sermon (which I delivered again for the cameras) in the first episode, turning me into a celebrity of sorts. I learned that the speed with which this happens can turn your head and change your world. ABC flew me to New York the week of the debut for a whirlwind publicity tour. For two days I got "the treatment." They provided me with a limousine, a driver, and a schedule jam-packed with more than 20 appearances, including *Larry King Live*, *The 700 Club* and *Good Morning America*. Backstage at *The Late Show with David Letterman*, I saw people fawning over stars like Justin Bieber and Ben Stiller—that kind of attention can change anyone's outlook. Frankly, it was flattering. When I returned home, I had 2,000 emails waiting for me. In the weeks that followed, hundreds of people from around the world called to say, "What are you doing? We've got the same problem here."

This attention tempted me to cross the line between modesty and self-promotion, making me think for a moment that I was *someone special*. Fortunately, I have a loving wife who was kind enough to caution me against that. Noticing my head had grown one size too large, one night Dee said,

"Remember, you're still Steve Willis, pastor of a small-town church." That brought me back to earth and still reminds me of my mission. I don't want to be a celebrity or promote Jamie Oliver—even though he is a talented, creative individual. My purpose is to spread the same passion that drives this renowned British chef: encouraging people to eat healthier so that we can all reap the benefits.

Christians love to talk about stewardship. Far too often, though, the discussion is restricted to money—usually to the giving of a tithe (a tenth of our income) to God's work. However, biblical stewardship encompasses much more, such as our time, talents and health. We are to treat our bodies with respect. We should eat to live, not live to eat. God gave us food to sustain life. Cramming ourselves with an overabundance of fatty meats, pizza, snacks and sugar-laden treats is not good stewardship. It is a prescription for disaster—especially when we combine that kind of eating with a lack of exercise, inadequate sleep and stress.

A Universal Picture

In his first letter to the Corinthians, Paul wrote, "Do you not know that your body is a temple of the Holy Spirit, who is in you, whom you have received from God? You are not your own; you were bought at a price. Therefore honor God with your body" (1 Cor. 6:19-20). The church's record in following these words is dismal. Far too many of us remain chained to the bondage of obesity, gorging ourselves on delicious goodies and exercising little restraint or wise *physical* stewardship. This behavior is every bit as careless as wasting our money, and in fact is often the cause of unnecessary health care expenditures. The Centers for Medicare and Medicaid Services expect U.S. health spending to increase at an average annual rate of 5.8 percent between 2010 and 2020. That means that in 2020, health spending will reach $4.6 trillion and consume nearly one of every five dollars spent.[8] Such staggering figures ought to alarm us.

Even worse, the people we should expect to lead the way are sometimes the worst offenders. Consider a report released in May 2010 as part of a seven-year, $12 million study at Duke University. Two researchers found that the obesity rate among United Methodist clergy ages 35 to 64 in North Carolina was close to 40 percent—10 percent higher than other residents—and that middle-aged clergy (both male and female) were diagnosed with diabetes, arthritis, high blood pressure and asthma at significantly higher rates than the rest of the population. Diabetes and other chronic ailments often translate into reduced life spans.

"The truth is we've got an epidemic in the United States," says Rae Jean Proeschold-Bell, an assistant research professor at the Center for Health Policy, Duke Global Health Initiative. "We didn't find, at this point, significantly higher rates of heart attacks. But unless these obesity rates are brought down, that is inevitable."[9]

Extrapolate from this snapshot of North Carolina's Methodist pastors and you have a glimpse of all denominations nationwide. The view from the pew isn't much better. A 2010 Northwestern University study demonstrated that religious people are slightly more likely than the non-religious to be obese.[10] However, whether it is moms or dads, brothers or sisters, Jews or Christians, rich or poor, nearly all American people groups are hooked on fast food, junk food and couch potato habits that are leaving us overweight, stressed out and dying too young.

Yet what is many pastors' reaction to this scenario? A seemingly insignificant story illustrates the problem. In the summer of 2010, I attended a pastors' luncheon but had to leave before it ended. One of our associate pastors remained and later related a joke another pastor had told after the meal. It concerned a minister who had died at the age of 60 from problems related to obesity. Twenty years later, two friends who had lived healthy lives before dying in their 80s showed up at the pearly gates. Greeting them with a wave of the hand, the minister smiled and said, "Good to see you. But I've been enjoying life up here for 20 years. What took you so long?"

The story prompted hearty laughter from most of the pastors there, but our associate pastor remarked, "It may have been good for him, but it wasn't so great for his family."

I know what he meant. My father's father died at the age of 64, primarily because he smoked two packs of cigarettes a day. I never enjoyed an adult conversation with him, because lung cancer took him away far too early. I sorely missed his presence at my high school and college graduations, as well as on my wedding day. I never had the benefit of his counsel during life's major transitions. I never knew the joy of seeing my grandfather at family gatherings and special occasions as I matured. Please hear the soft tone of my voice right now. You may think you're nobody special, and that nobody appreciates you. That is wrong and a self-centered way of looking at life. Many other people depend on you, admire you, and look to you for guidance, reassurance and love, even if they fail to express it.

Please know that overeating hurts more than our adults. Look at what it does to our children. According to a 2010 CDC report, childhood obesity is one of the nation's most prevalent concerns. The number of obese adolescents in the United States has increased by more than 300 percent since 1990. One study found that nearly 80 percent of children who were overweight between ages 10 and 15 were still obese at 25.[11] The CDC report pointed out that obese children and adolescents are targets of early and systematic social discrimination. The psychological stress resulting from this discrimination can cause low self-esteem and hinder academic and social functioning.

Eating isn't wrong. It's just that eating too much and choosing the wrong things is an abuse of God's good gifts. What I have discovered in leading our church to make changes in this area is that victory comes in small, almost imperceptible steps. Fried chicken still shows up at our potluck dinners, as do mashed potatoes and yeast rolls. But so do healthy salads, low-fat entrees and sugar-free desserts. Winning the food fight is a long journey that lasts for years—but it starts with a single step.

Setting an Example

Thanks primarily to Jamie Oliver's getting on the phone and calling a number of his friends, during the first phase of filming *Food Revolution* our church raised more than $100,000 needed to finish our family life center. We had already invested $1.3 million in the building, and we were committed to avoiding debt as we completed it. That final influx of funds enabled us to offer walking and exercise classes during the winter of 2010— which was one of the coldest, most bitter seasons I can remember. Without the center, we likely would have seen more backsliding in our fight for healthier living.

Although many churches aren't large enough to afford such facilities, they can still offer exercise classes or encourage members to seek them out. No matter what size the church, it can ask members to consider bringing healthier alternatives to its potlucks. Offering members wise guidance, scripturally based teaching, and the opportunity to alter their health habits is the best step pastors and church leaders can take. It generally isn't helpful to lecture members, browbeat them or speak on the topic too often. An overbearing emphasis can drive people away.

When it comes to promoting healthy choices, the most important thing every pastor can do is set a good example. That will take courage; as Proeschold-Bell noted in the Duke study, refusing to sample parishioners' pies, cakes or cookies runs the risk of offending them and provoking worse problems. I hope I don't come off as a frowning, judgmental, humorless prig. I still enjoy a good joke, cutting up with friends, watching football, relaxing with a good book, and taking family outings. I don't see foregoing eating meat. Occasionally, I will even eat a piece of fried chicken. However, there is a huge difference between occasionally enjoying a slice of pepperoni pizza and daily heaping unhealthy, calorie-laden choices onto our plates.

As we, as church and community leaders, attempt to inspire others, we must remember that many people will take two steps forward and one step back. Others will give up, either because they get too discouraged or because they are not willing to make tough choices. Remember, too, that doubters will seize on any failure as a reason to poke holes in our efforts or proclaim, "I knew it wouldn't work." Such comments usually reflect the speaker's failure or deep-rooted desire to maintain their chicken-wings-and-cheeseburgers status quo.

Although we still have plenty of parishioners who struggle with their weight, and some who joke that Jamie's show was a waste of time, today we also have people who once were anywhere from 40 to 80 pounds overweight and are now running distance races—and winning them. Five months after the mini-series aired, nearly 70 members competed in a 5K to raise funds for a local food pantry. Collectively we've lost more than a (literal) ton of weight. I am especially proud of Elizabeth Bailey. The wife of an Army reservist, she has lost more than 75 pounds. With faith, discipline and determination, she turned her situation and life around. Today she leads others to do the same.

We are one modest-sized church in a town of 3,500 just west of Huntington. Many people would label us ordinary—and that should encourage everyone who reads these words. People who think they need some kind of superhuman strength before they move forward aren't likely to change. Those who don't think their extra weight is that big a deal won't change much either. But those who have recognized the need and committed themselves to doing something about it have found success by following common-sense steps that come day by day. In the rounds that follow, I will outline a plan for change and suggest ways you can address the problems that face our nation. Whether or not you need to lose weight, this book will help you start on a healthier path that will bring healing to our land. Trust me—it's a whole lot deeper than a plate of food.

Remember that this book is training you for a fight. It will be a struggle. Just like in a 12-round heavyweight contest, each round will push you to reach new heights. Twelve rounds. That is what champions do. Don't throw in the towel and quit reading halfway through. Don't ever say, "I can't do this." Keep fighting.

As we move to Round 2, I am going to explain how I was called into the ring through a personal wake-up call that eventually revolutionized my thinking about food. God had to shake me up and make me realize that people dying before their time is not His perfect will. It all began with a poke in the belly.

Questions for Discussion

1. Do you think Jamie Oliver's producer calling the day after I asked God for help providing nutritional education to my congregation was mere coincidence or evidence of answered prayer? Have you ever had a similar experience?
2. Obviously the Huntington, West Virginia, area has a major health problem. What are conditions like where you live? Do you know the CDC statistics for your area? (If not, http://www.cdc.gov/obesity/index.html is a good place to start.)
3. Of all the statistics relating to the destructive nature of obesity, which stood out to you the most? Why?
4. What factors do you see as the most crucial in the modern obesity crisis? What are your first thoughts on how current obesity trends can be reversed?
5. When it comes to healthy eating, what do you think about the church's responsibility to set a good example?
6. How would you describe your feelings about your overall health?

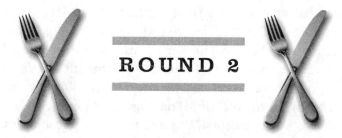

ROUND 2

Weighed Down

We were the worst. We just didn't know it.

Back in the fall of 2007, I flew to Dallas to visit an old friend from graduate school. Brad Payne had been an athlete at Pepperdine University. When we met in the mid-1990s, we became instant friends. We shared most of our classes, a love of sports, and a wild sense of humor that didn't fit the norm at Dallas Theological Seminary. Neither of us saw ourselves as future pastors. We came to Dallas to deepen our faith and hopefully find a way we could serve God, have fun, and make the world a better place.

Our school fees included an extra benefit: membership at the Tom Landry Fitness Center at the Baylor University Medical Center. Truth be told, Brad and I spent as much time at that gym as we did in class. Four or five days a week, we played water polo, shot hoops or pounded racquetballs—name a sport and we likely played it. We were in pretty good shape, with physiques to match. Back then, I never imagined that the effects of marriage, children, youth ministry and middle age would eventually settle over me.

When I got off the plane and joyfully greeted my old buddy, I immediately saw signs of *my* age in *his* lack of hair. Sure, I was developing some gray streaks along the top. However, since I still enjoyed a full set of follicles, I instantly thought of a Vin Diesel comparison to Brad's thinning pate. (I don't know what it is about guys, but millions of us find pleasure in making fun of one another's physical attributes. Ironically, I didn't notice that my friend looked as lean as he had in seminary). Before I could say anything, though, Brad stuck his index finger squarely in the center of my gut.

"My goodness, Steve," he said. "You've let yourself go."

The remark caught me off guard. I had always been tall and lanky, with a body more suited to basketball than grueling contact sports. For the first time ever, someone had insinuated that I was getting fat. I didn't know how to react. Granted, I was nearly 20 pounds heavier than I had been in grad school. But come on, man, *letting myself go?* Was he kidding? Back home in West Virginia, people often made fun of me for being so skinny. At nearly every church dinner, the ladies at the serving window piled extra-generous servings on my plate and admonished, "Steve, you don't look too good. You need to put on some weight."

Deciding Brad couldn't be serious, I let the comment slide. We went on to enjoy a fun weekend together. We went back to campus, saw some former professors, tracked down friends who still lived in the Metroplex, took in a professional basketball game, and visited some of our favorite restaurants—where I noticed that Brad usually didn't finish his meal. I wondered if he was suffering from digestive problems. All that good food, and he was leaving half of it on his plate! He didn't do that back in our younger days. Didn't he know there were starving children in Africa?

During my stay, we laughed at each other and life in general. The weekend left me with a strong impression: No matter how long it is between our visits, Brad and I will always be best friends. As he dropped me off at the airport for my return flight, Brad did something that best friends do. Pulling me away from other people so he could speak privately, he said, "Steve, really man, you need to work off that gut. It's only going to get worse once you hit 40. What are you going to look like in 10 years if you put on weight like you have for the past 10?"

Only a friend like Brad could make that kind of remark and not offend me. Still, I didn't take him seriously. I thought I was in good condition, particularly compared to other people back home. The way I looked at it, people around Dallas were a bunch of fitness freaks. Besides, between having three elementary-age children at home, coaching three different sports teams during the school year, working on my Ph.D., and ministering to 100 teens at church, I was pretty busy. An exercise regimen would have to wait for another day.

Another Wake-up Call

The following summer, I flew to Pismo Beach, California, to perform a friend's wedding. Dee and I went out a little early for a mini-vacation. For us, there is nothing like hiking out west. In our early years together, we had mounted Yosemite National Park's Half Dome, which calls for a 17-hour roundtrip hike to reach its 8,800-foot height. We had climbed Mount Moran, a breathtaking slice of the Rocky Mountains in the Grand Tetons whose flat-topped peak is just over 12,600 feet above sea level. Even when she was pregnant, Dee and I traversed a fair share of the Yellowstone Valley's 800 miles of trails.

We planned to cruise around Monterey before heading to nearby Carmel. There we would turn south and follow the Big Sur Highway that weaves along the California coast, creating stunning views that inspire painters, sculptors and just about every car commercial. Along the route, we planned to stop and hit a couple of moderate-to-strenuous hiking trails overlooking the Pacific Ocean. We were hyped! The driving went fine. The hiking? Rocky would have been disappointed in me. Halfway up the first trail, I felt so winded I had to take a 10-minute break after 5 minutes of wheezing. A runner, Dee didn't break stride. Naturally, I wanted to blame my short-winded efforts on the high altitude, but Dee humorously reminded me that since we were just a mile from the Pacific Ocean, I couldn't blame breathing problems on a lack of oxygen. "This isn't exactly hiking in the Rockies," she quipped, smiling as she left me in her dust.

At the end of the day, we arrived in Pismo Beach and went to the coast to watch the sunset over the ocean (a rare treat for someone from back east). As we sat there, I watched people cascading by us. Hundreds of sightseers were walking or jogging along the seashore. Others rode bikes. Some athletic types tossed balls or Frisbees. Everyone had one thing in common—they were thin. I felt embarrassed to take off my shirt and enjoy the sun. The spare tire around my waist had been developing for several years. For the first time, I was painfully aware that my body was out of sorts. Brad was right. I *had* let myself go.

As the sun dipped below the horizon, I asked Dee if she had noticed the physical condition of most of the people around us. Though she hadn't, once I mentioned it she agreed that they were much thinner than most West Virginians. We reflected on our travels to more than 20 countries and most regions of the United States. Neither of us could think of any place in the world where people were in as poor physical condition as in Huntington. "You know, it seems no matter what direction I travel from home, people get thinner," I told Dee. "I think we really have a problem." Little did I know how prophetic those words would prove to be.

A Blind Spot

Not long after we returned from California, our church made some staffing changes following a key pastor's departure. As a result, I started working with adults. After nearly 20 years of spending endless hours with teens—driving to their ballgames, counseling heartbroken 13-year-old girls who had just ended a two-week relationship with their dream guy, and cleaning up the vomit of teenage boys who thought chugging a gallon of milk in 30 seconds sounded like a good idea—I thought adult ministry would be a walk in the park.

Wrong! Within days of making this change, I received a call asking me to visit a close friend before his heart surgery. About 150 pounds overweight, he had battled high blood pressure for years. He was still relatively young, but in a recent examination his doctor had discovered blockages in a couple of heart arteries. Although we expected him to make a full recovery, I prayed with my friend and comforted his family. I had no idea that would be the last time we would ever speak.

Whoever thinks that life can't end in the blink of an eye has never stood in a hospital and watched a monitor flat-line. My friend survived the operation, but complications arose during surgery. A few hours later, doctors pronounced him dead. I was there when his heart stopped beating. I will never forget the look in his wife's eyes when the heart monitor beeped for the last time. Pain, regret and anguish flashed through dark pools, reminding me that as much as I would miss him, his family would be hurting much, much more.

As we left the hospital, we did our best to console one another. This was one of those times when I didn't have any soothing words to offer—no pastoral insights and no reassuring words from Scripture. After all, I was in shock myself. What do you say in times like these? "He's in heaven now" or "I'm sure he's in a better place" would ring hollow and might even provoke more sorrow or anger. Then a well-meaning family member uttered a phrase that changed my outlook and even my theological perspective. I'm sure that person was like me—digging to find words of consolation. This loving, caring family member said, "I guess it was just God's will."

Those words stopped me in my tracks. I knew this individual meant well, but I couldn't believe what I had just heard. It wasn't the time to preach, so I remained silent. Yet everything inside of me wanted to shout, "Don't blame this on God! It's not God's fault my friend is dead! If he had addressed his weight problem a few years ago, we probably wouldn't be having this conversation right now!" I didn't like thinking those thoughts about my friend. I felt like I was betraying his memory.

During the days leading up to the funeral, I experienced a full gamut of emotions ranging from anger to grief, sadness, loss and hurt—and then back to anger. *Why didn't he follow the doctor's orders? Why didn't he take better care of himself?* I was hurting for him, his family and myself. Don't misunderstand. My friend was a great man with many talents who contributed immensely to our church. He possessed a wonderful sense of humor, a deep love for his family, and a caring attitude that blessed people more than they likely appreciated during his lifetime. I loved him dearly. He just had this one blind spot—and unfortunately, it cost him his life.

On the evening of the funeral, our church was having a fellowship dinner. This night was potluck—the familiar smorgasbords that overflow with dozens of fine, home-cooked goodies. Each family brings a covered dish to share. With entrees and sides aligned single-file on tables, these dinners rival any buffet you can find at an all-you-can-eat restaurant. Fried chicken, pot roast, meat loaf, chicken and dumplings, mashed potatoes and gravy, macaroni and cheese, buttered corn, broccoli casseroles, biscuits and gravy, fresh rolls—you name it, we've got it. Oh, and the desserts! Mountains of pies; cheesecake topped with blazing red cherries; Frisbee-sized chocolate chip, peanut butter and sugar cookies; brownies, cobblers, and an assortment of cakes with cream cheese icing and other gooey frostings that would make any bakery proud. Dinners like these have gone on for years. The problem is that while we like to eat like our grandparents ate, we don't work like our grandparents worked. Modern labor-saving devices have spared us from lots of exercise. Too much, in fact.

After a short prayer asking God to bless the food to the nourishment of our bodies, we invited the older members to go through the line first. As they began to fill their plates, I stood at the end of the table and wondered exactly what we were doing to ourselves. We held these potlucks every month—and gathered for other feasts when there was a notable anniversary or other special occasion. I watched as people with sedentary lifestyles piled spoonful after spoonful of fattening foods high and deep. Though everyone laughed and enjoyed one another's company, I couldn't help wondering how many of these buffet lines my deceased friend had passed through. Had we played a role in the process that killed him?

Obesity's Real-life Impact

At the end of the evening, I headed back to my office to finish a little paperwork. As I turned the corner, I discovered a young couple waiting for me. As if on cue from God Himself, this couple told me they needed marital counseling. They didn't know what kind of day I'd had, nor did they know the person who had passed away, and I could tell from their body language that theirs was a pressing matter. So I sat and listened, struggling to pay attention to what at first seemed to be a litany of petty complaints.

The remarks I'm about to share are not simply this couple's story, but a composite of many similar scenarios. If I've heard this kind of sad story once, I've heard it a dozen times. Invariably, it winds down a road that ends in a statement like: "We're thinking we'd be better off to just go ahead and get a divorce."

Those words snapped me out of my mental fog.

"Divorce?" I replied. "You have several children together. Is it really that bad?"

For the next 30 minutes, the wife explained that they were struggling with a number of health issues, all related to obesity. The strain had taken its toll on their marriage. She was dealing with "Mom guilt" because when she got home from work, she was too tired to make dinner or help the kids with their homework. To make matters worse, her husband never helped out around the house. Financially, largely because they were going out for pizza or bringing home fast food five times a week, they had fallen behind on their utility bills. Plus, since her husband's insurance no longer paid for her diabetes medications, most of her paycheck went to cover medical expenses. (As an aside, if they decided to file bankruptcy, the government— meaning taxpayers like you and me—would have to pick up the tab.) They had reached the point where they were fighting constantly. Their kids reflected this chaos by acting out their frustrations at school, leading to discipline issues.

Then it was the husband's turn. He didn't have much to say other than to complain that they hadn't had any physical intimacy in three months, and he was sick of it. His wife had so many issues with her self-image that she had lost her sex drive. If this was a picture of the future, then he wanted out. Then he repeated the statement that had originally caught my attention: "We've prayed and prayed about this. Both of us feel the kids would be better off if we just split up and started over." This time, the words sent me over the top.

I am not an angry person. Anyone who knows me personally would tell you that I am one of the most fun-loving guys around. But on *that* day, I lost it. I didn't scream or raise my voice, but I said what I wanted to say. I usually temper my words a little, but not on *this* day. I told the couple they were blaming God for things that were not His fault. God did not want them to quit on their marriage, just as He did not want my friend to die. God wanted them to have an abundant life, just as He had wanted my friend to have a long, fulfilling life. However, too many marriages and lives were being cut short because of the pervasive sin of gluttony. This sin was affecting countless people—including the husband and wife sitting in my office at that moment—spiritually, emotionally, physically, economically, socially and mentally. The sooner they faced facts, the better off they would be. "God has a better plan for you," I said, the edge in my voice a bit too strong.

By God's grace, that couple forgave me for being a bit too passionate in the way I counseled them that night—perhaps because they knew that everything I had told them was the truth. Once they realized that most of their problems were related to their eating habits, they began to change. Their marriage improved, their finances straightened up, and they fell in love again. Over the next few months, I found myself counseling an increasing number of couples dealing with similar issues. I also realized I was visiting hospitals three or four times a week. It amazed me to see how much time got absorbed praying with people who wanted God to miraculously heal them, but who weren't willing to take any steps to improve their health.

I am not suggesting that visiting the sick is not an important part of a minister's role. Showing concern for people is one of the most important ministries Christians can perform. Yet, I chafed over the time consumed by driving to hospitals because of illnesses that were largely self-inflicted by poor nutritional choices. I'm sure other pastors can relate. Here are a few more productive things we could be doing with our time:

- Working with young parents to help develop their parenting skills.
- Doing more research to provide increased depth to our sermons.
- Cultivating leadership skills in our church officers.
- Reaching out with programs to help the poor.
- Meeting with other pastors and leaders for mutual encouragement and learning.

The ultimate result of widespread gluttony is that our families, workplaces, schools and churches lack the necessary leadership to advance in many areas that make the world a better place. The church's slovenly eating habits are literally costing it eternal impact. God is not pleased with such poor stewardship of our bodies, resources and time. Addressing this situation doesn't cost one thin dime (in fact, it will save us a few dimes). However, it does demand that we make an effort to change the status quo. If we want to win the food fight, we need to go on the offensive. Lying on the couch and gorging ourselves on potato chips is a sure way to lose.

The Man in the Mirror

The weeks following my friend's funeral were a struggle for me. Everywhere I went, I noticed the detrimental effects of obesity. Whether I was at the hospital, in church, at the grocery store or visiting local schools, I saw how people were suffering. Some struggled to make it up the stairs or squeeze into crowded elevators. I heard others wheeze as they walked into their doctors' offices. These were natives of my home state—people I loved and cared about. It felt like God was telling me I had to do something. I started with a look in the mirror.

While I wasn't obese, I couldn't escape the reality that I was overweight. People at our church would scoff at me for saying that, but according to every medical chart I found, I was nearly 20 pounds over my recommended weight. I started watching my caloric intake more closely and ran sprints with the sports teams I coached. Dee and I started taking brisk evening walks. Gradually, the spare tire around my waist deflated. I pulled on jeans I hadn't been able to wear in years. For the first time since my mid-twenties, I gradually lowered my weight to what healthy guidelines deemed acceptable.

During this time, any number of people expressed concern about my health or worries over my appearance. Nearly every day someone asked, "Are you feeling all right?" Rumors about my wellbeing started swirling, and some folks asked Dee if she had stopped feeding me. All I'd done was bring my weight down from overweight status to barely meet healthy guidelines, but people thought something was seriously wrong with me. Their reactions showed how skewed our perceptions have become.

Once I felt like I had developed a degree of faithfulness to wise eating and health practices, I knew I had to address the topic with our congregation. Yet, I didn't know how to go about it. Though I have never been one to shy away from discussing hot topics, speaking to people about their weight takes controversy to a new level. If I talk about the struggle with pornography, it is not as though everyone who deals with this issue has eyes that glow in the dark. If I speak about gossip, the guilty parties can't be identified by their flaming tongues. But if I broach the topic of gluttony, it is easy to see who struggles with weight issues.

God has blessed me with some incredible friends who serve as my advisors and overseers. I wanted to lean on their wisdom as to how to address this delicate subject. One evening, I called them together and shared my observations about how our area's plague of obesity was killing us, in more ways than one. Much like me when I was first confronted with the issue, they were not immediately convinced that obesity was all that serious a problem. They asked questions like, "Is it really that big of a deal?" and "Isn't there something else you should be preaching about?" and "Do you want half of our church members to get offended and leave?"

One of my dearest friends said, "Now, come on, Steve. It's not like someone is going to hell just because they're overweight." On that night, I could see that I was not going to automatically get their blessing to address the obesity epidemic among our people. We agreed to table the idea for a week—which wound up turning into six weeks. I couldn't fault them for their hesitancy to address this issue, though; it had taken me a year to face reality. I prayed that these guys would arrive at the same realization I had and help me in the cause.

Their delay actually proved beneficial, as it gave me an opportunity to face an issue I had to deal with personally—one more important than our struggle with poor nutrition and lack of exercise. My friend was right: People can be overweight and still go to heaven. No matter what else I write, please understand that whether you go to heaven has absolutely nothing to do with what you eat (see Matt. 15:11). Despite my passion about this topic, I can never forget that there is a more important, underlying principle.

There is a fundamental truth that God wants all of us to understand: There is nothing we can do to earn God's love or His favor. I struggled with this for a long time. We all have faults and failures, especially me. Until I understood this truth, I found myself constantly trying to impress God so that somehow I might earn myself a glorified reward in heaven. Then one day, a light bulb flashed in my head. I saw that whether or not I end up in heaven is not dependent on whether or not I am a smoker, liar, glutton, gossip, adulterer, or commit some other wrong for which others might harshly judge me. At the same time, my faith should help me over-come my struggles and lift me above my circumstances.

Balancing these two truths is like walking a tightrope with no safety net. It is quite a challenge. As I share about what our church did to touch our community, and how the publicity surrounding Jamie Oliver's series has created long-term results, I hope you will remember that no one in the food fight should get weighed down with guilt. If you are struggling in some area, whether your weight or something else, I do not want you to feel judged. In fact, if you are battling weight issues, it is not as if you need a book to tell you that. You already know. You may or may not be convinced about the seriousness of the problem, but you know you need to do something.

An important question to ask yourself is this: Are you trying to be good, exercise will power, and overcome whatever you struggle with for the purpose of earning God's favor? Or, are you doing it to impress the people around you? If you are trying to earn brownie points with God, you will fail and feel miserable. It is also unlikely that anything you do will gain that much approval from others. Be honest. How many times have you tried to lose weight? How many times have you fought the urge to eat one more bowl of ice cream? How often have you attempted to hold your tongue in an argument? Or to begin an exercise regimen? Or to stop smoking? Or to _____ (fill in the blank)?

Ultimately, while I hope to help other communities take steps to combat obesity, this book is not about weight loss, a special health care product, a cooking technique, or any other man-made program for im-proving your life. It is about finding a faith that helps you overcome your failures and lifts you above your circumstances. It is about the grace of God invading your spirit and compelling you to do what you can to help yourself and the community around you. I know many peo-ple who have found their way. I hope you do as well. As you go through this journey called life, understand that your health matters to God just like your prayer life, family life and church life. In fact, as we shall see, they are all related.

What Would Jesus Do?

Before you move on to the next round, will you take some time to notice the world around you? Can you see people whose eyes are creased into deep frowns, their faces wrinkled with worries, or whose steps are halting because they are literally carrying around so much weight? I never really "got" the problem with obesity until I took a few moments to observe those around me. Do this and you won't need a CDC report or the latest survey, news article or documentary. You will see the problem with your own eyes.

Occasionally I take friends to a fast-food restaurant, followed by a trip to a hospital. At both stops, I ask them to watch people entering and exiting the building. Then, based on these observations, I ask them to make a quick estimate. Based on the dozen or so people they've just seen, what percentage would they say are struggling with dietary issues? When I do this, we generally arrive at an estimate of 60 percent or higher. See what number you come up with.

I tell folks that if they want to get a good look at the way most Americans live, they should hang out at the emergency room for an hour or two. That will give them a much better picture of reality than just looking at their immediate friends. It is easy to while time away in middle-class suburbia, where people generally have enough income for gym memberships and organic produce. When we do this, we can forget that the masses are straining just to pay their bills and put meals on the table. The sad thing is that we have created a system where it is cheaper for people to fill their plates with fatty foods than with fruits and vegetables.

As someone who tries to live according to the principles of the Bible, I cannot ignore the fact that Jesus hung out with the masses. He didn't live in the suburbs, surrounded by highly educated people who read books just for pleasure. If He were on earth today, He would be waiting with the people in the emergency room or providing food for the folks who order off the dollar menu (not to mention those who don't even have a dollar). To get an understanding of our nation's peril, maybe we all should do a little more of the same. Once our church started developing a perspective like this, things began to change.

Stepping into the ring requires an awareness of the reasons for the fight—a knowledge of why it is even important that you lace on the gloves. If you are ready, prepare for Round 3.

Questions for Discussion

1. When you run into old friends, do they make comments about your weight? Do you perceive their remarks as loving or judgmental? Why?
2. Have you ever received a wake-up call alerting you to the need to tackle a physical challenge? Describe what action you took.
3. Have you or a friend suffered the adverse effects of too much weight? After reading Round 2, how do you look at that situation?
4. Do you think a healthier lifestyle would improve your close relationships? Why?
5. In the past, have you made attempts to make lifestyle changes, only to encounter a lack of support from those closest to you? How did that affect your success?
6. In what ways have you tried to impress God? Why do you think we go to such great lengths to impress Him, even though the Scriptures tell us He loves His children no matter what?
7. Over the next few days, observe the lifestyles of people in your community. Record your observations and share them with a few other community-minded people.

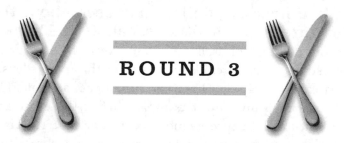

ROUND 3

Does God Really Care?

A few years ago, I heard Dr. Bill Brown, president of Cedarville University, deliver a speech about the impact of culture on our attitudes, beliefs and behaviors. He pointed out that each of us, like a fish in a vast ocean, is surrounded and influenced by our culture. We see *everything* through its lens. Try as we might, we cannot escape it. Those who believe they are not affected by their culture are simply unaware of its impact. In fact, those who are oblivious to their culture's influence are more likely to be controlled by it. As a result, they will be unable to rise above it, becoming little more than drones in society's hive.

Such is the battle when it comes to the power that food exerts over American society. I accompanied Jamie Oliver to his pre-*Food Revolution* appearance on David Letterman's TV show. As Jamie discussed his efforts to alter Huntington's eating habits, Letterman ridiculed the idea that people could change, and scoffed, "It will never get better." (To Letterman's credit, he later invited Jamie back to the show and apologized for his negativity.)

I cannot accept this attitude. If I didn't believe that people have the ability to change, I would leave the ministry. It is easy to get cynical about this fallen world, but the key to leading change is staying positive. You must embrace hope. If you are convinced something is right and is God's will, you must have faith that He can bring it about. Ultimately, faith changed my perspective and the perspective of our church's leaders when it came to publicly addressing the congregation's obesity epidemic.

Risking the backlash that might result from confronting those you love is a demonstration of genuine care. (As opposed to selfish love, which is worried about keeping people happy and therefore won't broach any topic that might prompt anger.) Any good parent knows the feeling. Sometimes children unknowingly or unwisely make poor choices. While they may not enjoy the chill they'll have to endure for the next few days, parents who love their children will warn them about the consequences of foolish decisions. A friend says, "You have to love them enough to let them hate you for a while."

Addressing the Problem

Driven by love, I was ready to risk speaking about our congregation's problem with obesity. That brought me to a Wednesday night in August 2008 and the final step before writing the sermon that would later be featured on Jamie Oliver's mini-series. Several weeks earlier, the men gathered in my office had told me I was crazy for raising this issue. Now they were praying with me for a cultural change. They asked God to make a difference in people's lives and open their hearts to the truth. Afterwards, our oldest leader said, "We know you need to address this. Just make sure you do it with a feather and not with a hammer."

I would like to tell you that I left that meeting brimming with confidence—that I believed God would perform a miracle and lives would change. The truth is, I was scared to death. Now that the elders had given me the go-ahead, the reality of what I was about to do weighed heavily on me. How was I going to communicate this problem? What illustrations would I use? How would people respond? I remarked to my wife that this sermon might very well be my last.

As I scrambled to put together an outline, it struck me that the only evidence I had to prove that we had a major health problem was anecdotal. Every city has people who struggle with their weight. Just saying "we have a problem" seemed inadequate. I needed hard-core evidence. A few days before that Sunday, I found it. I awoke to a front-page headline in Huntington's daily newspaper proclaiming our area the unhealthiest in the nation. The story about the CDC report cited government statistics to support my contention. As I had surmised back when I was on the beach in California, Huntington was indeed at the heart of the fattest region in America. Now I had proof.

I felt excited, not because of our lack of health, but because I believed this was the wake-up call our community needed. Surely now people would take responsibility and make the necessary lifestyle changes to improve their health. Wrong! Although this study headlined TV news that evening, stations didn't discuss the report's serious implications or our need to change. Most interviewees cited socio-economic discrimination or complained that this was another attempt to poke fun at West Virginia. Local health care providers proclaimed the study faulty. I don't remember one individual going on camera to agree with the report. As has often been said, "Denial ain't just a river in Egypt." I guess it is just the nature of human beings to respond to criticism by employing defense mechanisms.

Since my first reaction when confronted with my own protruding belly had been to deny I had a problem, I couldn't judge the folks in our area for their resistance to the truth.

Despite the uproar, I knew the CDC was "spot on." While I had no idea whether or not the Huntington area was the worst in every health category, there was no question we were in dire straits. At this point, I had all the ammunition I needed. Sunday morning couldn't come quickly enough. Now it was just a matter of communicating the truth in a way people would understand and accept.

Culture Shock

As Dr. Brown pointed out, any good teacher will recognize the impact that culture has on his or her students. Effective educators will utilize aspects of societal influences to communicate ideas in such a way that students can move from the known to the unknown. For example, if I wanted to teach a group of teenagers about the importance of respect, I would ask them to discuss the ramifications of Kanye West's rant against Taylor Swift during the 2009 Video Music Awards. (If you ask, "Who is Taylor Swift?" you aren't too connected to teen culture.)

When addressing my congregation about obesity, I applied this principle by calling on the biblical example of someone who possessed an incredible understanding of how culture affects one's ability to learn: Saul of Tarsus—or, as he is better known in Christian circles, the apostle Paul. I call Paul the best cross-cultural communicator the world has ever known. He had a pedigree similar to that of Dr. David Kessler, the physician I referenced in Round 1 whose stellar résumé runs about 10 pages long. Were he alive today, Paul could lecture at Harvard on the foundations of natural law, visit Wall Street to discuss economic theory, and then hop down to Washington, DC, to deliver a homily about the evolution of our constitutional republic. Afterwards, he could board a plane to Rome for a theological exchange with the Pope, followed by a political debate in Moscow on the causes behind the fall of Communism. Did I mention that he would speak each country's native language?

Keenly aware of Greco-Roman culture, Paul faced a challenge when it came to communicating an orthodox view of Christianity. The problem stemmed from remnants of a Greek society influenced by Plato's teachings and elements of the heresy that later became known as Gnosticism.

In short, this society viewed the human body as negative. They saw the world through dualistic eyes, believing that lesser gods created the physical. To them, that meant the mental and spiritual aspects of humanity represented the race's sole redeeming quality. Because of this worldview, many Greeks thought Jesus was a mere spiritual apparition. In their minds, God would never come to earth in the form of human flesh, since that would contaminate His spirituality.

Dualists separated life's physical aspects from the mental, emotional and spiritual. They reasoned that since the body was destined for the grave, it was evil and counterproductive to one's ability to develop the most important aspects of humanness. This thinking influenced most first-century religious groups, including those with ties to Christianity and Judaism. The more unbalanced views divided into two extreme camps:

- People known as ascetics would punish their bodies, attempting to deny the flesh any semblance of pleasure. They would starve themselves, cut themselves, or deprive themselves of sleep and sexual fulfillment. Ascetics abstained from just about any behavior that might gratify the natural or material self, hoping to suppress urges conflicting with their spirituality.

- At the other end of the spectrum, the forerunners of Gnosticism believed that since the body was fallen and separated from the soul, they possessed a free license to satisfy fleshly cravings: Eat, drink and be merry, for tomorrow we die. From their perspective, it didn't matter what they did *to* or *with* their bodies as long as they thought positive thoughts and did no harm to their fellow man.

So the apostle Paul arrived on the scene, fully aware of the dualistic philosophies embedded in Greek culture. However, instead of opening with theological guns blazing, he recognized the positive aspects of the people's religious beliefs. Whether in Athens, Rome, Asia Minor (modern-day Turkey) or Jerusalem, Paul, being a good teacher, took his audience from the known to the unknown. He didn't attack their culture or religious background, but found something positive and started with that.

Examples of this practice appear in Paul's letter to the people at Colossae. First, he affirmed their belief that humanity's intellectual and spiritual dimensions were its most important aspect. The opening sections of the epistle include several references to the Colossians' intellectual growth: "We have not stopped praying for you and asking God to fill you with the *knowledge of his will* through all *spiritual wisdom* and *understanding*. And we pray this in order that you may live a life worthy of the Lord and may please him in every way: bearing fruit in every good work, *growing in the knowledge of God*" (Col. 1:9-10, emphasis added).

In other words, Paul was saying, "You're right: The intellectual and spiritual aspects of our identity are indeed the most important facet of our humanness." But then Paul comes back with a right hook—a culture shock. He proceeds, over the next few paragraphs, to refer to the body in positive terms. In addition, he emphatically states that Jesus came in bodily form (see Col. 1:15-24; 2:9-11) and instructs this licentious group to stop their drunken orgies or God will judge them harshly (see Col. 3:5-7). Can you imagine the Colossians' consternation? Paul was proclaiming that the body was good, and that what they did with their bodies mattered. He wrecked dualism. According to his teaching, they could not separate who they were physically from who they were spiritually, intellectually or emotionally. Paul was saying, "Yes, it makes a difference. God does care about how you use your bodies."

Bought at a Price

Paul's assault on dualism extended beyond the Colossians. To the people in Corinth, he wrote the words I quoted in Round 1: "Do you not know that your body is a temple of the Holy Spirit, who is in you, whom you have received from God? You are not your own; you were bought at a price. Therefore honor God with your body" (1 Cor. 6:19-20). If you grew up in church, you may have heard this passage before. What you need to grasp is the radical nature of this statement to a group accustomed to abusing their bodies. *You mean God really cares about what I do with my body?* many in his audience likely thought. *Come on, Paul. Are you serious?*

"Absolutely," Paul would have replied. "We must understand that our bodies are more than flesh and blood." To paraphrase 1 Corinthians 3:16, Paul would have said, "Our bodies not only house our souls, but also serve as temples for God's Spirit!" This is why taking care of our physical bodies is such an awesome spiritual responsibility. Do you understand the profound nature of this assertion? Paul taught that God's Spirit lives inside each of us. Not only do we bear His image, but we also carry Him with us wherever we go. Our bodies facilitate God's presence in our homes, workplaces, schools and communities. A loving, eternal, all-powerful God chooses to get carried around by a bunch of weak human beings. It is not that God *needs* us for transportation; He *chooses* to operate this way. Paul declared that the blessing of having God inside us includes a notable responsibility.

Paul made another point that deserves great emphasis. Various schools of thought rightly observe that our fleshly cravings can lead us to make selfish decisions. That much is obvious. I don't know about you, but I have never heard a toddler say, "You know, I'm pretty hungry right now, but I'm going to be patient because Mommy needs a nap and Daddy is really busy." No, from the time we are born, if we humans want something, we let everybody know it until we get some satisfaction.

Our toddler-like habits carry on into teen life. Even now, as I watch my own children advance into this stage, it amazes me to see how sweet, gentle, fun-loving young people morph into selfish brats when they haven't had enough sleep or a snack in the last 90 minutes. What is it about the unsatisfied flesh that brings out the worst in us? When our perceived needs aren't met, self-preserving behavior seems to come naturally.

That is the problem. Selfishness *is* natural. We are born selfish—and the more we feed our flesh, the more it drives us to indulge it. One of my graduate school professors once said, "The only reason young babies and old men seem so godly is because the former group has yet to acquire the skill to demonstrate their sinful nature and the latter group is losing it." Just look around you; observe how nearly every TV commercial appeals to selfish desires. Something is wrong with the human condition, and the human race isn't making it much better. All this selfishness does not make God happy. On the contrary, as a righteous and fair judge, He is angered by it. Some people don't like the idea of a God who gets angry, but when I think about the alternative, I will take the God of the Bible every time.

To illustrate my point, I'm going to ask you to think of someone you love. Now, imagine two thugs break into that person's house and abuse him or her, almost to the point of death. After the police capture the perpetrators, and the thugs go on trial, you pay a visit to the courthouse to see what kind of punishment these criminals will receive. The jury returns a "guilty" verdict, and the judge brings the convicted men before him. As he opens his mouth to speak, your loved one grabs your arm. Then the judge exclaims, "I know you men are guilty, but I love you both. I've always loved you. Therefore, there will be no fine and no jail time. You are free to go."

What would you think? Would you say that judge is fair? Truly loving? No, you would want justice. A good judge does not let crime go unpunished. At the least, someone should have to pay a hefty fine—the more serious the crime, the larger the fine. When it comes to the crime of selfishness, we are all guilty. We have all lied; we have all lusted after something that wasn't ours. If we're honest, we will admit that we have stolen a thing or two in the past. We are a bunch of lying, coveting thieves. Into this selfish world, God sent His Son to pay our fine. When Paul said that we were bought at a price, that price was Christ's life. When God says our bodies belong to Him, we cannot overlook the price He paid to redeem them.

Honor God with Your Body

Once we understand the price Jesus paid, we can see why Paul told us to honor God with our bodies. He doesn't want us to go on like spoiled children, always making selfish choices. He wants us to mature, discipline ourselves, and use our physical bodies for good. This theme recurs throughout Scripture. Consider the following statements and their integration of the physical into our Christian discipleship:

> May God himself, the God of peace, sanctify you through and through. May your whole spirit, soul and *body* be kept blameless at the coming of our Lord Jesus Christ (1 Thess. 5:23, emphasis added).

Clearly, Paul, in giving equal billing to the physical and spiritual, refuted the claims of dualism. God wants us to dedicate the totality of our being—not just part of ourselves—to Him.

> So whether you eat or drink or whatever you do, do it all for the glory of God (1 Cor. 10:31).

When is the last time you visited a pile-it-high buffet and thought, "How will God be glorified by what I put on my plate?" For that matter, how much thought did you give to what you drank at dinner last night? Did your beverage help your body function in a healthy way? Do your other daily choices honor God? In contrast to the culture of his day, Paul exhorted his friends to make wise dietary decisions—because how we eat and drink matters to God.

One of my favorite verses in the Bible is the climactic statement of Paul's letter to the Romans. In chapter 12, verse 1, Paul pulls together the thoughts of the previous 11 chapters: "Therefore, I urge you, brothers, in view of God's mercy, to offer your bodies as living sacrifices, holy and pleasing to God—this is your spiritual act of worship."

Leading up to this point, the apostle had delivered one of the best—if not *the* best—theological perspectives in human history, assuring his readers that by God's providential hand, and through the merciful work of Christ, they could find freedom from the sin that enslaved them and then live freely for eternity. In view of what God had done on humanity's behalf, what did Paul say He expects? A follower of Plato would argue we should dedicate our minds to God's worship. A romantic would encourage us to give God our affections. Some would argue that the soul comes first, and that we must give God full devotion of our spirits. Yet of all the aspects of humanness Paul could have mentioned, he urged readers to present their *bodies* as living sacrifices.

The term Paul uses for *body* has far-reaching implications. The Pauline concept of yielding our bodies involves more than just giving God control over our fleshly desires. When we sacrifice our bodies to God, we are giving Him absolute devotion in every aspect of our lives.

In light of Paul's admonition, when was the last time you went to the health club thinking, "This is my spiritual act of worship"? What about pushing away from the table before you are stuffed? Or getting a good night's rest? All these are in essence spiritual acts, but we have somehow moved away from seeing our bodies as an integral part of honoring God. What we do *with* and *to* our bodies matters. Stewarding them is not just something to do when we find time. We must develop our physical selves just like we give emphasis to our emotional, spiritual and intellectual development. These aspects of our humanity cannot be separated from one another. They are inextricably connected.

Paul wasn't the only biblical author who addressed the importance of taking care of the body. Moses delivered countless directives regarding proper dietary choices for Israel. Nearly all the verses of Leviticus 11 and Deuteronomy 14 describe the best sources of protein. There are hundreds of passages dedicated to personal hygiene and dietary commands.[1] Going back even further, what was God's first gift to Adam and Eve? He placed them in a garden with *every* fruit-bearing plant and vegetable necessary for proper nutrition (see Gen. 2:8-9).

Christ's words also demonstrate that our health matters to God. When asked to identify the most important command in Scripture, He replied, "Love the Lord your God with all your heart and with all your soul and with all your mind and *with all your strength*" (Mark 12:30, emphasis added). Do you see the totality of this command? We cannot just love God emotionally (heart), spiritually (soul), and mentally (mind). He wants our physical strength as well.

Failing to commit our bodies to God spells trouble—as it did for that overweight couple I mentioned in Round 2. They had committed their hearts, souls and minds to God, but their marriage sputtered because they had not committed their bodies. They could not love God with all their strength while they carried around an extra 100 pounds. Ingesting a steady diet of garbage had caught up with them. Thankfully, they came to the realization that God didn't want just 75 percent; He wanted their all. Likewise, if you are not giving Him control of your body, it is impossible for you to fully serve Him. Jesus came that we would have a full life, but the devil came to steal, kill and destroy (see John 10:10). One way that the world's negative forces destroy life is by influencing us to make poor dietary choices.

Making Children Suffer

Your dietary choices are not just about you. It is one thing when adults pay the price of bad nutritional choices, but another altogether when those choices affect our children. Unfortunately, as I mentioned in Round 1, our children are suffering greatly due to our lack of oversight. I cannot imagine that this makes God happy. Extra weight literally slows children down, makes them the target of ridicule from cruel classmates, and damages their health.

Have you ever tried to swim with a weight belt around your waist? I did that once in a lifesaving class. Fifteen extra pounds caused me to sink straight to the bottom of the pool. The instructor said even the strongest swimmers cannot handle that kind of extra poundage. I remembered his comment a few years ago, while on a tour of Israel. As our group stood beside the Sea of Galilee, I noticed a large round stone sitting atop a perch of rocks just yards from the shore. The stone looked to weigh between 75 and 100 pounds. When I asked the guide why it had been placed in such a prominent location, he said it was an old millstone used for crushing wheat seed. Then, he referred to the Scripture where Jesus said, "Whoever causes one of these little ones who believe in Me to stumble, it would be better for him if a millstone were hung around his neck, and he were thrown into the sea" (Mark 9:42, *NKJV*).

Jesus' point? Do not make choices that will hurt His children. The societies, churches, families and schools that harm children will have a mighty price to pay on judgment day. Without question, faith and fitness intersect at this crossroads. Faith demands that we protect children by giving them the nutrition, education and exercise opportunities necessary for healthy physical, emotional, mental and spiritual lives.

The Sin of Sodom

If I asked you, "What was the grievous sin that caused God to destroy Sodom and Gomorrah," what answer would you give me? I've asked this question to a hundred people who grew up in church, and every one of them gave me the answer, "Homosexuality." I broach this sensitive subject because I feel it is important for us to understand the relationship between the "sin of Sodom" and the subject of this book. Yes, God eventually destroyed Sodom and Gomorrah for their grievous sins, but the book of Genesis never directly states which sins. The typical reader of the book of Genesis sees the evidence for homosexuality in those ancient cities and often deduces that because that sin was present, homosexuality must have been the primary reason for God pouring out His wrath on them.

However, the Bible never says that. In fact, the prophet Ezekiel tells us exactly what was the sin of Sodom, and he minces no words in his explanation: "Now this was the sin of your sister Sodom: She and her daughters were arrogant, overfed and unconcerned; they did not help the poor and needy. They were haughty and did detestable things before me. Therefore I did away with them as you have seen" (Ezek. 16:49-50).

There it is! Do you see it? Sodom's sin was pride, gluttony, and apathy toward the poor and needy! God destroyed them because they overfilled their bellies with food while the poor and needy among them were starving—and they didn't care! What could be more indicative of our nation? We are dying from eating too much while thousands die from eating too little!

We'll talk much more about the world's nutritional disparity later in the book, but for now I want to ask this question: Why are the sins of homosexuals so grievous to the American Church while we tolerate the sins of gluttony and malnourished children within our own camp? As Jesus asked,

"Why do you look at the speck of sawdust in your brother's eye and pay no attention to the plank in your own eye? How can you say to your brother, 'Let me take the speck out of your eye,' when all the time there is a plank in your own eye? You hypocrite, first take the plank out of your own eye, and then you will see clearly to remove the speck from your brother's eye" (Matt. 7:3-5).

Change Your Mind

Since the Bible commands us to use our strength to honor God, serve others and protect children, this begs the question: Why isn't the Church doing more to improve our world's physical wellbeing? The simple answer is that we have allowed Platonic, dualistic and Gnostic philosophies to creep back into our belief systems. Why else would pastors joke about killing themselves with food? Why else would they preach against hate, envy, pride and sexual sin but forego messages about the gluttony that is destroying millions of lives?

Like modern-day Gnostics, we have separated the physical from the spiritual, seeing no connection between physical indulgence and spiritual failure. It is like declaring, "God can have my heart, soul and mind, but how I eat and exercise is none of His business." (Few Christians would verbalize such a statement, but their lifestyle choices proclaim it for them.)

One caution here: Although we must be responsible about how we treat our bodies, it is possible to value one's physique to the detriment of mental, emotional and spiritual health. Balance is necessary. Some folks spend hours in the gym and never touch fattening foods. Yet their self-image is so wrapped up in their bodies that they forget about spiritual development or cultivating their minds and emotional wellbeing. I have counseled many physically fit people who are as emotionally drained as the obese. Life is not about improving only one aspect of ourselves. The physical is important, but who we are on the inside outweighs appearances (see 1 Tim. 4:8-9).

Remember, too, that no matter what our weight or health condition, each of us is engaged in a spiritual battle. In his letter to the church at Ephesus, Paul admonished, "For our struggle is not against flesh and blood, but against the rulers, against the authorities, against the powers of this dark world and against the spiritual forces of evil in the heavenly realms" (Eph. 6:12). His point? Our fight is not just about physical realities. The mental and spiritual precede the physical.

There is a correlation between these elements. When we let ourselves go mentally, we are prone to get out of shape physically. Our mental outlook influences our physical choices. People often turn to comfort food because of emotional emptiness. Some think that going through a drive-up window four times a week isn't that big a deal. Others believe they cannot do any better; defeat in the mind usually precedes defeat in the body. If we are going to change our diet and exercise habits, we must first be convinced in our hearts and minds that we need to change. Otherwise, when things get stressful or inconvenient (and they will), we will lapse into our old ways of thinking, eating and acting. When that happens, we are down for the count.

Fire in My Bones

I recently read an online comment from a nationally known pastor who said that we can work out all we want and eat low-fat salad dressing and we are still going to die. While what he said is true, do we really need to be so fatalistic? Is that the message the most obese nation in the world needs to hear? Just because we're all going to physically die some day, does that mean we should abuse our bodies by failing to work out and eating full-fat, ranch-style dressing?

I believe that at the heart of this fatalistic mindset is a profound lack of respect for the elderly population. We increasingly live in a society that does not value older people. Our movie stars seem to get younger and younger, and barely anyone on the Billboard Top 40 charts today is over 40. It's as if people over 40 lose the ability to act well or produce good music. There is something about our culture that tends to undervalue the acumen of those who are advanced in years.

How does this relate to the food fight? For the most part, eating poorly doesn't take you out of the mainstream of life in your 20s and 30s. It starts slowing you down in your 40s and 50s, with the effects of a lifetime of poor nutrition manifesting themselves fully around 60. So when people make snide remarks such as, "Well, you're going to die from something," in essence they are saying, "It's not a big deal if I die early."

In our church, it is no secret how much the senior citizens contribute to our various ministries. I cannot explain how important it is for these godly grandparents to be around for their grandchildren. One thing I can say for sure is that some of the most powerful characters in the Bible accomplished their greatest deeds after the age of 60. Moses and the parting of the Red Sea, Joshua and the walls of Jericho, Daniel and the Lion's Den . . . the list goes on and on. All performed heroic acts after their AARP cards came in the mail! What would the world have looked like if Moses had died of heart disease when he was at the ripe old age of 75? Sadly, we are losing thousands of quality individuals in their 60s—not because they die from natural causes, but because they did not take care of their bodies during their earlier years.

As I said earlier, to win my food fight I first had to change my thinking about food. That changed my outlook and actions. Nowadays, I find myself relating to the prophet Jeremiah. A passionate prophet who loved his people, Jeremiah felt a calling to speak out against his day's social ills. He had a burning inward drive to speak on God's behalf: "But if I say, 'I will not mention him or speak any more in his name,' his word is in my heart like a fire, a fire shut up in my bones. I am weary of holding it in; indeed, I cannot" (Jer. 20:9).

In the summer of 2010, when *Charisma* magazine deemed me "the apostle of health," at first I felt embarrassed. However, it has become a label that I am willing to wear. I am not a prophet by any biblical standard, but when it comes to proclaiming God's justice, defending children and advocating for the poor, I do have "a fire in my bones." I have no choice. It has to come out! Sometimes that gets me in trouble, but I would rather live this way than aspire to draw a paycheck, retire and take a pension for a few years before I die.

At the same time, I am nothing special. I am just a small-town pastor who grew tired of watching people die too early. I can't sit by while children are prevented from reaching their full potential because we as adults and community leaders aren't willing to make the sacrifices necessary to teach them proper nutrition. Many other people have this fire in their bones as well. Jamie Oliver has it. Elizabeth Bailey has it. Over the next few rounds, you will meet others who feel the burn as well. Do you feel an inner spark? One thing I have learned in this life is that people who have a fire in their bones get things done. Fan that flame!

A Call to Action

I don't want to condemn other pastors, leaders or church members for committing a sin I was once guilty of myself. In fact, our church heeded the challenge of tackling poor nutrition and a lack of exercise much better than I did. Clearly, the Spirit of God was at work. Not only were our church members not upset with me after my sermon on obesity, but also more than 60 people immediately enlisted in a program designed to help them lose at least 40 pounds. They embraced the fact that God is a God of second chances.

The reaction of our congregation demonstrates an important principle: Once we leave the realm of ignorance, we bear a greater responsibility. As James 3:1 warns, "We who teach will be judged more strictly." Now that we are enlightened, it is a different matter. If you see the harrowing statistics and scriptural mandate to change, yet refuse to do anything, I do not want to be next to you when you stand before God someday.

If I sound a little upset about the Church's silence, good. But please understand. I am not a little upset. I am extremely upset! In the eighteenth century, many in the Church led the way to secure our rights as a constitutional republic. In the nineteenth century, many worked to fuel the abolitionist movement that eventually ended slavery. In the twentieth century, many marched on Selma, Alabama, and Washington, DC, to promote civil rights. But in the twenty-first century, where is the Church on this fundamental issue of getting proper nutrition to the masses? People are dying by the millions, the poor are being exploited, and many of our children don't have a fighting chance. Rise up, Church. Your people need you!

The Rules

I graduated from East Bank High, the same school that produced the legendary Jerry West. Young people who weren't around when he led West Virginia to the NCAA championship game and the Los Angeles Lakers to new heights can check out the National Basketball Association's logo. That is West's silhouette. Before Michael Jordan or LeBron James came along, Jerry was arguably the best player in the history of the game.

Between the years when West was on the team and my playing days, our high school program deteriorated a little—actually, a lot. From the time I was in sixth grade until my sophomore year in high school, East Bank won a total of four games. We also lost respect for our program, our coach, and the game of basketball itself. The summer before my sophomore year, the junior varsity coach encouraged me to attend a weeklong basketball camp. Since my chances of making the team were about 50-50, I signed up. When I arrived, Jerry West was there. I couldn't believe it!

After a few hours of working on fundamentals and shooting drills, he pulled our team aside. He talked about respect for the game, giving our all, and representing our families and school with pride. As he concluded, our JV coach walked over. Pointing at him, West said, "The key to you all winning again is directly related to your ability to live by Rule #1 and Rule #2." He then held up his index finger and explained, "Rule #1: The coach is always right. Rule #2? Anytime you think the coach may not know what he is doing, refer to Rule #1."

Before you read further, it is important that we establish our Rule #1: *We have to change the dietary culture in the United States.* When distractions come your way, when the David Lettermans of the world proclaim that this is a fight we can't win, when the task seems too large, when the pounds aren't coming off, or when things just seem to keep getting worse . . . refer to Rule #1.

I am doing my best to inform, sadden, inspire and motivate you. I may have angered you—and if so, I'm glad. If watching your friends and family members die needlessly doesn't upset you, what I have to say won't matter. If being part of a culture that encourages obesity in a shocking number of children doesn't make you chafe, you will remain part of the problem. If seeing people waste their God-given lives doesn't light a fire under you, I don't know what else to say.

After several years of fighting this battle, I have found that people who pay lip service to the obesity epidemic are of no help at all. They do more harm than good. They tell you to keep up the good work, and then return to joking about their clogged arteries. Don't judge them too harshly; I once did the same. However, to make a difference, we cannot wait for everyone to catch the vision. This is a food fight. It will get messy. We are swimming upstream against a torrent of opposition. Those who aren't committed to the fight will simply "go with the flow."

If you are like me, your blood is boiling. You feel a righteous indignation that is compelled by love. You have to *do something.* You may not be sure what, but by God's grace, you will act. Keep on reading and you will get plenty of ideas as to how you—yes, YOU—can bring about lasting change. Whether it is individually or in your family, church, community, school or political system, you are going to do something. Taking action lines up with Rule #1. Continue to Round 4 to read about the legendary historical figure who altered his university's food culture.

Questions for Discussion

1. How do you see the impact of culture on your philosophical outlook on life in general? How about on your attitude toward food?
2. Was David Letterman right when he scoffed at the idea that people can change? Why do so many people concur with him when it comes to the obesity epidemic?
3. Discussing obesity from the pulpit was risky business. Is it just in church that raising this topic meets with resistance, or is it considered taboo in other forums as well?
4. In regard to discussions of obesity in our society, what extremes do you see on both sides of the issue?
5. In what ways do you see the philosophies of dualism infiltrating the Church? How about our society in general?
6. How are you passing on your eating habits to your children? Is this a good thing or a bad thing?

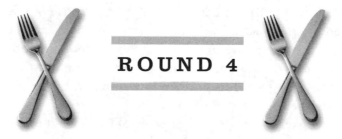

ROUND 4

A Biblical Plan
for Change

Nearly 3,000 years before Jamie Oliver filmed his award-winning mini-series in Huntington, a different fight over deficient school lunch programs took place. In the seventh century BC, a few young men found themselves at the center of a battle over their government's flawed system of nutrition and education. After confronting the powers-that-be—in an almost miraculous turn of events—these teenage captives revolutionized the diets of hundreds of students in the ancient world.

Many have likely heard the biblical story of Daniel in the lions' den, or some variation of it. Yet, they probably don't know much else about one of the foremost prophets in the Hebrew Bible. Likewise, many may have heard of Shadrach, Meshach and Abednego standing against the king of Babylon and consequently facing a fiery furnace. What fewer people realize is how all four of these young men forged their hearts of courage in the flames of their school lunch lines.

In 605 BC, King Nebuchadnezzar's armies marched into Jerusalem and laid siege to the Holy City. "Then the king ordered Ashpenaz, chief of his court officials, to bring in some of the Israelites from the royal family and the nobility—young men without any physical defect, handsome, showing aptitude for every kind of learning, well informed, quick to understand, and qualified to serve in the king's palace. He was to teach them the language and literature of the Babylonians. The king assigned them a daily amount of food and wine from the king's table. They were to be trained for three years, and after that they were to enter the king's service" (Dan. 1:3-5).

These orders represented a common practice in ancient times. When a country invaded and conquered another, it forced the best and brightest of the defeated nation to use their skills and gifts to benefit the conquerors. In effect, Nebuchadnezzar took the valedictorians from Jerusalem's high schools and gave them a full scholarship to Babylon University. In exchange, he demanded a lifetime of service. This cohort of conscripted servants included Daniel, Hananiah, Mishael and Azariah. Each carried a deeply religious name symbolizing their commitment to Yahweh, the God of Israel.

As if it weren't enough to take these young men away from family and homeland, the Babylonians subjected them to thorough indoctrination, including refusing to let them keep their given names. In their place, Babylon substituted names reflecting pagan deities: "The chief official gave them new names: to Daniel, the name Belteshazzar; to Hananiah, Shadrach; to Mishael, Meshach; and to Azariah, Abednego" (Dan. 1:7). To cap this terrible turn of events, these handsome young men were castrated to eliminate any chance they would form relationships with females in the king's palace.

Formulating His Plan

Poor Daniel. One day he is rich, handsome, and one of the best and brightest students in Israel. The world is his oyster. One week later, his family is dead, he will never return home, and he has lost his manhood. Sure, he is living in the king's palace with full access to the king's rich buffet, but Babylon has vanquished his childhood hopes and dreams. How would you handle such a crushing blow? Would you consider your life ruined and meaningless? Would you be too demoralized to resist your captors' commands?

The next part of this story catches my attention. In spite of all that had happened and the stunning reversal of his fortunes, Daniel had the resolve to look over the king's food and say, "No, thanks" (see Dan. 1:8). I'm sure most of the other Hebrew teens tried to make the best of a bad situation by assimilating into the culture. Not Daniel. The Babylonians could change his name, remove his ability to father children, and immerse him in an ungodly culture, but he still refused to eat meat sacrificed to pagan gods. Determined to be faithful to his God, Daniel took a series of steps that, at any moment, could have led to his execution. Instead, God used his courageous spirit to change an unhealthy food system that was detrimental to everyone involved.

When it comes to transforming our food system, we can follow Daniel's steps for making a change:

Step 1: Make Up Your Mind to Be Different
Before I say anything else about Daniel, it is worth reiterating a point I made in the previous round: If you don't make up your mind to change your culture, your culture will change you. Daniel resolved to be different,

not to fit in, and to take the necessary steps to change. Since he didn't exactly live in a democracy, that decision was terribly risky. Yet this teenager wanted to be distinct from those around him. Are you:

- Struggling with your weight?
- Running the rat race like everyone else and often whisking your children through the drive-up window for dinner?
- Needing to break years of poor nutritional habits?

You must first make up your mind that you want to change—that you *need* to change. I'm not talking about mere behavior modification, but an attitudinal change. This isn't just about being thin. It is about being healthy and seeing your children eat well, live well and love well. You must want to be healthy physically, mentally, emotionally and spiritually, and be willing to do whatever it takes to move toward those goals. You can't be willing to settle for anything less. Like Daniel, you must resolve to take this step.

Step 2: Seek God's Grace

If making up our minds to be different were enough, most of us would already be healthy. However, "ye olde willpower" is not enough. No one wants to be fat and out of shape. Most of us have tried to get in better physical condition or change bad eating habits—often with only marginal or even negative results. Left to our own devices, most of us will fail. The apostle Paul endured this battle. In his letter to the Romans, he described caving in to the desires of his flesh: "I do not understand what I do. For what I want to do I do not do, but what I hate I do" (Rom. 7:15). A few verses later he added, "For I have the desire to do what is good, but I cannot carry it out. For what I do is not the good I want to do; no, the evil I do not want to do—this I keep on doing" (vv. 18-19).

If you have dieted, you understand these verses. Although you want to eat healthier, you go out and consume three servings of chocolate fudge and hate yourself for doing so. Somewhere inside is the desire to do the right thing, but you CANNOT carry it out. There is a big part of you that wants to quit, but for some reason, you just CANNOT do it on your own. It is the thing you hate the most that you keep on doing. Welcome to reality. We cannot win this fight on our own. The problem of poor nutrition and obesity is so dreadful that no one person or group can turn it around. We need God's grace and favor.

The solution appears at the end of the passage in Romans, where Paul asked, "Who will rescue me from this body of death?" and then answered his own question: "Thanks be to God—through Jesus Christ our Lord!" (Rom. 7:24-25). Paul's wrestling match illustrates that God's favor is not something we deserve. Nor can we earn it. Through no effort of our own, He chooses to help us. That is grace. When someone does us a favor, it is not a favor if they are paying us back. It is only a favor if we didn't deserve it. This is what makes grace—as *Amazing Grace* author John Newton wrote— truly amazing.

The more I think about it, the more I realize how God shed His divine favor on our church throughout the *Food Revolution* process. On a worldly scale, what are the odds of Jamie Oliver's producers hearing about us? Yet God brought an entire film crew to our small, rural state and told our story to the world. The producers found it in their hearts to drum up more than $100,000 worth of labor and materials so we could complete our family life center and have our town's finest kitchen facility. Though the show's finale featured only a few seconds about the center's completion, Jamie and his friends generated more donations for our church than all the other projects on the show combined. That is the favor of God.

We see this same divine favor on Daniel. God softened the heart of the "school principal" so he would listen to Daniel's request to change his lunch menu. This authority figure had no logical reason to listen to the snotty-nosed foreign teenager's request. Besides, as the story goes, he had nothing to gain and everything to lose by cooperating with Daniel's proposal. "I am afraid of my lord the king, who has assigned your food and drink," he admitted. "Why should he see you looking worse than the other young men your age? The king would then have my head because of you" (Dan. 1:10).

However, something funny happens when God gets involved in human affairs. People agree to do things they otherwise would never have considered. Kings give you gifts. Health gets restored. By His gracious hand, God renews hope. If you are struggling with your health, will you pause for a moment and seek the grace of God? Will you humbly ask for His favor? Whatever you are looking for, if it is something great, you will need His grace to obtain it. Before moving to the next step, consider what God would have you do. Seek His grace.

Step 3: Develop a Plan

If Daniel had simply stood up and declared, "I'm not going to eat any more of this pagan king's food," they likely would have chopped off his head before he finished the sentence. Instead of speaking disrespectfully to the king's officers, Daniel wisely had a plan when he mentioned his desire to revolutionize the king's deli: "Please test your servants for ten days: Give us nothing but vegetables to eat and water to drink. Then compare our appearance with that of the young men who eat the royal food, and treat your servants in accordance with what you see" (Dan. 1:12-13).

There are a few things worth noting here. First, Daniel's plan was *specific*: He would follow a vegetable and water diet for 10 days. He knew exactly what he wanted to do and for how long. Second, he had a method for *measuring success*: The water drinking/vegetable-eating group would be compared to the "control group" of wine drinking/meat-eaters at the conclusion of the experimental period. All successful plans are specific and measurable. You must have objective goals before starting your journey, and you must have a mechanism to measure success. Some people say, "I want to lose 20 pounds," but their only plans are walking more and eating less. That is not specific enough.

I know something about planning because, early in my ministry, I found myself burning out trying to come up with creative ideas for weekly youth group meetings. One summer, I received a miraculous inspiration. Instead of waiting until the Monday before the meeting to come up with discussion topics, I scheduled them a year in advance. I sat down with other leaders and brainstormed about what we needed to teach during the coming school year. Then we planned ways to incorporate those teachings over the next 36 weeks. This revolutionized my creative process. No more aimless wandering through lesson plans. Some people fear that being organized and planning ahead would limit their creativity. I found the opposite to be true: Putting a structure in place ahead of time actually allowed me to become more creative—as well as to find greater joy in my work. By planning and organizing, I actually became more creative.

The same principle applies to eating. If you wait until 3 o'clock on a Tuesday afternoon to think about dinner, you are in trouble. Chances are you will end up getting rushed and heading out to eat fast food. However, if you plan meals in advance, you give yourself the opportunity to shop more wisely, cook more wisely, and spend more wisely on your nutritional choices. The key to life change is developing specific, measurable goals and *planning a timeline* by which those goals can be achieved and evaluated.

I do not know why, but many faith-based folks see planning as an indication of a lack of faith—they think they should just "follow the Spirit." On a theological basis, I respectfully disagree. The parameters for how we are to live must stem from the attributes, characteristics and behavior of the God we seek to emulate. Why should I love others? Because God is love. Why should I not tell a lie? Because God is truth. Why is murder wrong? Because God is life. Why should I be committed to my spouse? Because God is faithful to me. A proper understanding of self should find its foundation in a proper view of our Creator.

Consequently, if we are created to reflect the image of God, how can we be anything other than a planner?

- When God created human beings (see Gen. 1-2), He clearly had a plan for what He was going to do and how He was going to do it. He even had a planned-out job description for Adam and Eve (see Gen. 1:26).

- When God called Moses to lead the Hebrew children out of Egypt, He had a plan to free the Israelites from their masters (see Exod. 3:6-20).

- Note the words God spoke through the prophet Jeremiah: "For I know the *plans* I have for you . . . *plans* to prosper you and not to harm you, *plans* to give you hope and a future" (Jer. 29:11, emphasis added).

- Jesus knew the Father's plan for His life. He repeatedly told His disciples that He had to go to Jerusalem in order to be crucified, buried and resurrected (see, for instance, Matt. 16:21). Ultimately His life fulfilled the plans God had spoken through the Hebrew prophets.

Since God was, and is, such a great planner, it should come as no surprise that Noah followed a plan in building his ark, Ezra and Nehemiah planned the rebuilding of Jerusalem, Paul planned numerous missionary journeys, and Solomon planned to build the great Temple. Can you imagine Solomon undertaking his Temple-building project with no plans? That would have been a disaster. Like it or not, you are working on the temple known as your body. Do you have a specific, measurable plan? Or have you aimlessly done a little bit here and a little bit there? Like the architects of old, you need a plan for success. As Solomon wrote, "Commit to the LORD whatever you do, and your plans will succeed" (Prov. 16:3).

I can hear you protesting: "I don't know how to come up with a plan" or "I've had plans before but they failed." Later, I will discuss in detail how to make good plans to revolutionize your health. In the meantime, I should alert you that I have seen even some of the best-laid plans fail because they didn't incorporate the next step.

Step 4: Enlist Help for Accountability and Support

Solomon's wisdom also applies to this step: "Plans fail for lack of counsel, but with many advisers they succeed" (Prov. 15:22). If you have repeatedly tried and failed to improve your health, I would suggest that your initial plans likely did not include both the *advice* of those knowledgeable in exercise and nutrition AND *accountability* to those who value healthy behavior. Simply stated, winning the food fight demands accountability and support. You need God's help and the help of those around you.

I don't know if Daniel had wisdom beyond his years, or if he just, like most teens, wanted to do everything with his peers. Either way, notice how he enlisted the support of friends after coming up with his plan. Earlier, I cited verses 12-13, where he suggested that a few of the young Israelite students be allowed to eat only vegetables and drink nothing but water for 10 days. Either Daniel was quite a persuasive leader, or these other young men loved him dearly. They literally placed their lives on the line to help Daniel succeed. We all need people like Hananiah, Mishael and Azariah—close friends or family members who will lay aside their own agendas to support us. These are the kind of people who are willing to go through a new eating plan with us and live side by side with us during our struggles—folks who will go to the gym with us, run an extra mile, or meet us three days a week for a brisk stroll through the park.

This is why Solomon wrote, "Two are better than one, because they have a good return for their work: If one falls down, his friend can help him up. But pity the man who falls and has no one to help him up! Also, if two lie down together, they will keep warm. But how can one keep warm alone? Though one may be overpowered, two can defend themselves" (Eccles. 4:9-12). Two are always better than one:

- If you fall down (literally or figuratively), a friend will pick you up and not let you quit. There is power in a friend. Better yet is a group of friends who work out together and push one another to excel.

- If you lift weights, you need a spotter. Plus, if you have someone pushing you, you will try harder.

- At home, cooking for two is cheaper (per person) than cooking for one. You can take turns cooking, and it takes half the effort to prepare healthy meals for the entire family.

Like Solomon, I pity those who fall and don't have anyone to help them up. I don't know many people who can win the food fight alone. If you are in a church where no one seems to care about healthier living, no one is interested in keeping you accountable to a workout regimen, and the pastor doesn't think taking care of your body matters to God, you may want to find another church. Yours is not preaching the whole counsel of God (see Acts 20:27). I tell our people I am willing to err on the side of caring too much and pushing a little too hard. Many pastors are more worried about offending people than they are about defending them from things that will literally kill them. Of course, issues like this call for walking a fine line—a pastor can easily cross it and get in someone's face. Still, when it comes to our health, God has called us to keep one another accountable.

As I said previously, with children sometimes you have to love them enough to let them hate you for a while. We all know parents who lack the will to tell their kids, "No." I have struggled with this myself. Instead of pushing our children to do better, it is easier to give in to their demands or ignore their inappropriate actions. But God wants more from us as parents—and as members of His Body. So go to your pastor or church leaders and ask them to help keep you accountable to getting healthier. Remember, you have made up your mind to be different, and you want to be successful. Part of achieving success comes from finding three friends who love you enough to let you hate them for a while (but only a short while).

However, don't stop with those three friends. Like Daniel, each of us needs a "chief official." This is someone who will test us, measure us, and kick us in the behind if we don't meet our goals. Unlike Daniel, who was under Babylon's authority, you need to give this person permission to act as your trainer. Sometimes you may not like this individual, because he or she will not let you quit. You must tell your trainer at the outset that failure is not an option. That way, if your trainer sees that you are not making sufficient progress, he or she will intervene and help you adapt.

Ask your closest friends and family to read this "step 4" section with you. Have your church leaders read it as well. You need their help, and they need to hear you asking for help. Winning the food fight takes a team effort.

When I lived in Texas, people used to tell a story about one of my favorite First Ladies, Barbara Bush. (This story fits into the category of urban legend, but it makes a good point.) As the story goes, at that time her son, George W. Bush, was an executive with the Texas Rangers. Her husband, George H. W. Bush, was president of the United States. As the president's motorcade traveled to a Rangers' baseball game, they stopped at a gas station for a restroom break. When President Bush emerged from the restroom, he noticed Barbara talking to a station attendant—an older man. President Bush noticed how friendly the attendant and Barbara seemed. As they parted ways, the two embraced.

After climbing into the presidential limousine, the somewhat jealous president asked Mrs. Bush, "Who was that man you were talking to?"

"Aw, George," she said in a slight drawl, "he was just an old boyfriend from my high school days. I haven't seen him in 40 years. Come to find out, he's the owner of that gas station back there."

The president smiled with pride and quipped, "Well, Barbara, what do you think about that? If you had stayed with him, you'd just be the wife of a gas station attendant."

"Don't flatter yourself, George," she quickly responded. "If I had stayed with him, HE would have been the President of the United States."

Don't underestimate the power of a supportive spouse.

Likewise, remember the power of a supportive family. Occasionally, I work with families who have a loved one coming home from an alcohol rehabilitation program. I impress on family members that if they want the recovering addict to succeed, they must commit to keeping their home alcohol-free. Even if they don't have a problem, they voluntarily relinquish their freedom to drink for the good of the person who struggles with alcohol. I advise them to stop going to clubs or restaurants that overtly serve liquor. In all but one case, family members willingly took these steps. The family that disregarded my advice saw the recovering addict relapse within two weeks and spend three more months in rehab.

Similarly, if someone is trying to break free of food chains, family members need to be considerate of that person. In the same way a family must remove beer and wine for the sake of a recovering alcoholic, a supportive family will rid their home of their loved one's food weaknesses. In our house, a bag of Doritos won't last longer than 15 minutes, because my sons like them so much. Consequently, we only buy them on *rare* occasions. Likewise, a side of beef in a shark tank would last longer than a carton of ice cream lasts around my teenage daughter. My soft spot? A tasty breakfast would consist of an entire box of Fruity Pebbles. Different family members struggle with different kinds of unhealthy foods.

I find it interesting that when Jesus gave us the model prayer, He didn't ask the Father to help us deal with temptation. He didn't say, "Strengthen us when we are tempted." Rather, He wisely stated, "Lead us not into temptation" (Matt. 6:13). In other words, get the unhealthy food out of the house! This kind of precaution characterizes how people in our health movement have succeeded. Those who are winning the food fight have also followed the pattern I just outlined:

- They were part of accountability groups.
- They participated in a team effort instead of trying to work their plans on their own.
- Almost every one of them had a "chief official" whom they respected and didn't want to disappoint.

By contrast, those who refused to reveal their weight to others, whose self-consciousness would not allow them to open up to an accountability partner, and who refused to submit to a "chief official" usually relapsed back into their old ways. They struggle to this day.

Step 5: Practice Self-control and Persevere

One might think that once Daniel enlisted the support of three friends and a chief official, he had almost completed the job. After all, he had accomplished four of the five steps of success, right? No, Daniel's vegetable-and-water plan only marked the beginning of the hard work. For the next 10 days, everyone's life was on the line. I am sure their stomachs longed for the king's buffet. They likely thirsted for a small goblet of grape juice or some other sweet nectar—anything but bland, lukewarm water. Looking over the gooey, sweet desserts on the table, thoughts of *Oh, if I could have just a nibble* likely entered their minds.

As hard as it must have been to abstain from these choice delicacies, I can imagine that dealing with their peers' taunts and emotional abuse was equally difficult. Can't you see the four teens at the dinner table, facing ridicule as they chewed on a celery stick instead of a nice side of beef? I am sure they heard such comments as, "Do you think you're better than us?" or "Don't judge us because we're eating this way." It seems to be a constant of human nature to resent those who try to be different.

Expect similar reactions if you get serious about changing your diet. The saddest part of my journey has been the negative response of some of those close to me, including family members. Others in our church who were trying to get healthier faced similar opposition. Friends in the community and extended family members didn't understand what we were doing and took offense at our new routines. Without any of us saying a word, they felt judged. To a certain extent, we did offend them.

This is where we have to be careful about how we treat others. If we condemn them for their lack of knowledge and understanding, in essence we are judging ourselves, because we too once had a similar state of mind (see Rom. 2:1). We must make every effort to carry ourselves in humility and love those around us who are still overcome by our culture and slaves to their own desires. The best way we can improve ourselves and set a good example for others is by demonstrating self-control and perseverance. The apostle Peter writes, "For this very reason, make every effort to add to your faith goodness; and to goodness, knowledge; and to knowledge, self-control; and to self-control, perseverance; and to perseverance, godliness" (2 Pet. 1:5-6).

Did you notice the order there? We start out with *faith* that, by God's grace, we can do this. We have the desire to do that which is *good*. Next, we educate ourselves in the *knowledge* of healthy nutritional choices and exercise. Still, we then have to practice *self-control*. We know going into this battle that it is going to be a fight, so we must make good choices daily and *persevere* until we reach our goal. Reaching our goals and fulfilling our plans is an act of *godliness*. God is a planner who succeeds. In achieving success by His grace, we become more like Him.

The Fruit of Self-discipline

As we practice self-control and persevere, good things will start coming our way: "At the end of the ten days [Daniel and his friends] looked healthier and better nourished than any of the young men who ate the royal food" (Dan. 1:15). Don't you look forward to that day? I am talking about when other people start noticing how your body is changing. The day when your friends say, "Man, are you losing weight? How are you doing it? You look GREAT!"

I know we aren't to do things for others' praise, but it feels good when people in our lives recognize a job well done. When we start getting compliments, though, we must remember to give the glory to God. It is only by His grace that we are able to accomplish any good thing. As we give Him honor, He will honor us (see 1 Sam. 2:30) and use our success to make the world around us a better, healthier place.

Notice what happened to the school lunch program at Babylon University. Once the official saw that these young Hebrews' diet made them healthier than everyone else, "The guard took away their choice food and the wine they were to drink and gave them vegetables instead. To these four young men God gave knowledge and understanding of all kinds of literature and learning. And Daniel could understand visions and dreams of all kinds. At the end of the time set by the king to bring them in, the chief official presented them to Nebuchadnezzar. The king talked with them, and he found none equal to Daniel, Hananiah, Mishael and Azariah; so they entered the king's service. In every matter of wisdom and understanding about which the king questioned them, he found them ten times better than all the magicians and enchanters in his whole kingdom" (Dan. 1:16-20).

God blessed Daniel and his friends for their obedience. It was no accident that these men, who were the healthiest physically, also became the healthiest mentally and spiritually. You cannot separate the physical from the spiritual. Honor God with your body, and He will honor you in more ways than you can imagine. You may have picked up this book hoping to lose a few pounds and find tips for healthier living. Once you start winning the food fight, you are going to find victory in other areas of your life. As you continue reading, pray about some God-sized goals. Think bigger than you have ever thought before. Allow God to inhabit every aspect of who you are, so that as your body starts to change, you will change the world around you. I believe with all my heart that God will do this. The key question is: Do you?

In the upcoming rounds, you will hear from people who have found success, people who have failed, and people who initially failed but eventually found success. My hope is that by sharing various people's stories and methods, I can arm you with knowledge that will help you design specific, measurable plans and enable you to win the food fight. In the process, I hope to see our indulgent culture break the chains that have a chokehold on our children, our churches, our communities, our schools and our nation. However, as you get ready for Round 5, remember that change begins with you.

Questions for Discussion

1. What sensations do you experience when you stand before a buffet brimming with rich foods? How can you empathize with Daniel and his friends?
2. What do you anticipate will be the most difficult aspect of "being different" from people around you?
3. When it comes to good health, what does it mean to seek God's grace?
4. Have you tried unsuccessfully to lose weight? Describe the plan you followed and why it didn't work.
5. Do you have a support group that can hold you accountable for good health practices? If not, where can you find one?
6. What foods tempt you the most? How many of those are around your house right now? What steps can you take to see that they are removed?
7. Do you think you will have support at home? Why or why not? How can your family or others close to you assist you in your attempts to get healthier?

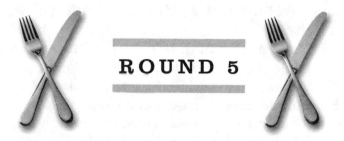

ROUND 5

The Man in the Mirror

The crowd of 250 teens at the statewide youth camp chatted excitedly as they waited for *American Gladiators* star Valerie Waugaman to take the stage. Even though it had been a couple of years since she had appeared on network television, her "Siren" persona lived on via the Internet. Many of these teens had probably fantasized about being one of the amateur contestants who matched muscles with the show's gladiators. Of course, if they actually tried taking on this buff body builder, they would likely wind up like potatoes in a food processor. I can tell you one thing for sure: I wouldn't challenge her.

Once Valerie climbed onto the platform, she held the attention of kids who are easily distracted by their electronic gadgets. She demonstrated some feats of strength and then turned the conversation to the importance of healthy living. The teens cheered her wildly as she shared her message. Their enthusiastic reaction to her exhortations left the unmistakable sense that they were ready to shout, "Yeah, we're going to do it!"

Seizing the moment, Valerie smiled and said, "Here's my first challenge for you." She paused as the buzzing reached a fever pitch. "For the rest of this week, stop drinking pop."

Pow! You could feel the air escape from the room with the force of a punctured hot-air balloon. I could sense the collective "aww" reverberating through their minds. Their sudden silence hinted at unspoken questions: "What? You want us to give up our Mountain Dew? We can't drink Coke? What are we supposed to do when we order pizza? Drink water? You have got to be kidding. That just isn't realistic."

We can chuckle over youthful enthusiasm turning to mass dejection when those teens recognized the price of walking the road toward better health. Yet, is that much different from how we behave as adults? When it comes to implementing a plan to reverse their bodies' deterioration, most folks are missing in action. While those who weigh 100 pounds or more above their ideal weight would proclaim their eagerness to lose it, how many are willing to exercise 30 minutes a day? How many will trade in their sodas or high-calorie energy drinks for water? Few will commit to paying the price even when it comes to such minor lifestyle changes.

But that is what it will take for our area to shed its unhealthy label. The same is true of our state, the two states bordering the Huntington area (Ohio and Kentucky), and America as a whole. We can talk all day about national initiatives, grand designs and sweeping reforms, but change starts on an individual level. A church that is thriving and seeing new people follow Christ is made up of a bunch of individuals demonstrating His love and telling others about Him in daily life. Likewise, a community that registers healthier statistics is the outgrowth of a number of individuals deciding to change the ways they eat and exercise. Thinking otherwise is like expecting a boxer who climbs into the ring without any gloves on to win the fight.

The Pain of Change

Change will never take place until the pain of staying the same is greater than the pain it takes to change. As the old adage goes, you have to be "sick and tired of being sick and tired." This is what Rick Ball discovered once he passed age 40. After being prescribed a number of medications for dizziness and high blood pressure, Rick was sick of being fat and out of shape. He could remember his younger days of playing baseball and basketball. He had been active in our church's intramural leagues through his early thirties.

When his sons started playing sports, he stopped playing so he would have time to drive them to all their games. Through it all, Rick kept eating the way he had when he was running up and down the basketball court. As a result, his waistline spread wider and wider until he tilted the scale at 250 pounds. He dreaded running into old friends or acquaintances, since that often prompted the question, "You've gained some weight, haven't you?"

"I couldn't do anything," recalls Rick, the general manager at a successful trucking company. "It took my breath away just to get out of bed. I felt horrible. I was wearing pants that were extra tight because of my weight, and big, loose T-shirts that wouldn't reveal how heavy I had become. I would come home after work and eat dinner, then take a nap for an hour and still go to bed at 10 o'clock. It snowed one night, and it took me an hour and 15 minutes to shovel out the driveway because I had to stop and rest so much. I used to be able to do it in 30 minutes. I said, 'This is it.'"

Rick realized the reasons he had offered to justify his constant weight gain were just excuses. He had made statements like, "Well, I'm past 40 now and it's time to gain weight . . . you know, this is something that is just to be expected . . . Shoot, I'm not so bad. Look at other people my age; they weigh even more." Ironically, even as he tried to rationalize his ever-increasing size, Rick never felt comfortable with such justifications. Deep down inside, he knew he had strayed out of line.

Recognizing that he couldn't keep eating the same way and expect to lose weight, he went online to research nutrition sites. Rick learned that dinners laden with potatoes and pasta dishes promoted his creeping bulge. Leaving those and other fatty choices behind, he switched to a diet featuring more chicken, fish and vegetables. He also started walking a half-mile on the treadmill every morning before work. Gradually that became a mile. Three months later, he had moved past three miles and could jog for half the distance. When the inside routine began to bore him, he switched to walking outside.

Rick also noticed that his job, which involved large amounts of paperwork, required him to sit behind a desk for much of the day. Seeing how walking helped him slice nearly 50 pounds from his frame, he started looking for more ways to exercise at work. Instead of hopping in a car to drive the short distance to the truck lot to see customers, he started walking. If someone called from the maintenance department, Rick walked over to see them. During lunch breaks, he made a point of walking around the property. Adding this to a two-to-three-mile routine at home at least four times a week has helped him maintain his weight loss since 2006.

Soon, his wife, Shelley, joined him in his health kick. This provided an additional boost. Although she didn't need to lose as much weight as he did, her willingness to eat the same things (Rick is the cook and grocery shopper in their house) made it much easier for him to maintain his plan. Instead of chowing down on a plate of biscuits and gravy before leaving for the office, he would fix an omelet made with vegetables. At night he cut out fatty steak, or pot roast and potatoes, in favor of lean meats and vegetables.

Rick and Shelley also held each other accountable. When they went out for dinner, she started encouraging him to order water instead of Coke. If he leaned toward old favorites like garlic mashed potatoes or Cajun-style pasta, Shelley would ask, "Are you sure you want to order that?" After thinking about the weight he had dropped, Rick would change his order to something like a healthy chicken breast served with beans and rice. He had learned the value of resisting gravy-drenched mashed potatoes or a baked potato smothered in butter, sour cream and bacon bits. Such additives are so familiar they sound like part of a normal diet. Yet they are the kinds of substances that contribute to America's caloric disaster.

Although Rick and Shelley still like to eat out, they have learned many tricks of the restaurant trade. Fortunately, they had family members who managed outlets of well-known national chains. These relatives alerted the couple to numerous ways the restaurant industry uses sweets, fats and salts to get us to crave their "food experience." Rick and Shelley's son (who has since left the industry) assisted me with my research for this book by filling me in on a number of behind-the-scenes processes through which food providers intentionally prepare their food to stimulate overeating. "Our goal was to get you used to eating large portions so that it took more and more money to get you full," he told me. "If you aren't stuffed when you leave our restaurants, we haven't done our job. If a couple is going to spend $50 on a meal, they want to feel like they got their money's worth." He went on to share with me that employees get perks and bonuses for "upsales," the casual dining equivalent to super-sizing. The more a waiter or waitress sells high-profit appetizers, such as cheese fries and potato skins, the better the perks.

Most of this probably comes as no surprise to you. After all, restaurants are businesses and of course want to make money. I just don't know that we consider exactly *how* they make their money. When it comes down to brass tacks, selling foods with the highest profit margins is the quickest way to make a buck. Restaurants aren't mainly concerned with how much money you spend. They would rather have you pay $5.99 for potato skins that cost them $1 to produce ($5 profit) than $6.99 for shrimp dip that costs them $4 to produce ($3 profit). The unofficial motto is: "Make it as cheap as you can, as fast as you can, so you can get them in and out as quickly as you can." This philosophy leads to high quantities of customers but low-quality foods.

The restaurant industry doesn't make billions of dollars a year by accident. They know exactly what they are doing when they organize their menus, their seating arrangements, the music they play, the lighting in the room—everything is designed to manipulate your behavior in ways that will render them the most profit. Unfortunately for their customers, the foods that make them the most profit are also the foods that make us the unhealthiest. Dr. David Kessler (the Harvard-trained doctor, lawyer and medical school dean I mentioned earlier) recognized this problem and began wondering what the relationship was between his own weight issues and eating out. What he discovered is pretty scary.

Sugar, Fat and Salt

In *The End of Overeating*, Kessler describes how foods laden with sugar, fat and salt (the cheapest foods to produce) temporarily alter our brain's chemistry in ways that compel us to overeat—hence the idea of appetizers.[1] From what I can gather, it is no accident that humans are made this way, for foods containing sugars, fats and salts provide quick energy to the person who needs it.

I don't know about you, but when I'm in a bad mood, all my wife has to do is whip up some Italian food and miraculously I feel fine. Similarly, have you ever noticed that when you are sick, you start feeling better when you eat? I sure do. Well, the reason we are like this is that God designed us to think and feel this way. When we do something that helps us survive as a people—whether it is food, sleep, sex, or anything else necessary for the propagation of our species—motivational pathways in the brain reinforce that particular behavior. When we participate in a primal behavior, various chemicals are released in the brain that momentarily make us feel better, both physically *and* emotionally. Once we've experienced the behavior that leads to a positive physical and emotional response, we begin to crave that feeling again, which drives us to a number of other behaviors in order to obtain another stimulating response. For example, when a young man is physically attracted to a woman, "ain't no mountain high enough, ain't no river wide enough, ain't no valley low enough" to keep him away from his woman!

One study demonstrated this principle ever so powerfully with regard to our primal need for food. Food was placed at the far end of a room with an electrified floor between the subject animals and the food. If the animals wanted the food, they had to walk across the floor to get it. Even when the animals hadn't been fed for a while, the shock of the floor kept them from progressing any further to obtain the food. Dr. Kessler observes that under normal circumstances, hunger did not provide sufficient motivation to act—because of the negative consequences. However, when scientists stimulated the reward centers in the animals' brains, even the animals that had eaten recently were willing to get shocked all the way across the floor to obtain more food.[2]

Have you ever felt this way? You are not alone. Each time we eat certain combinations of sweets and fats, or salt and fat substances, endorphins are released in our brains, giving us a euphoric feeling. (These substances truly are emotional "comfort foods.") This was God's way of rewarding a behavior necessary for survival. It programmed our ancestors to eat as much high-energy food as they could, whenever they could—because they didn't know when they would get to eat again. This natural, God-given desire to eat foods loaded with sugars, fats and salt can rise to a level only slightly lower than the breaking point for cocaine when there is a pattern of overstimulation.[3] (This explains why we sometimes feel "addicted" to certain foods!)

Sometime in the last 30 years, restaurants figured out they could maximize their profits by tapping into these primal needs. Some national restaurant chains go as far as using needles to inject extra grams of fat and salt into chicken. As a result, even though you think you're getting a healthy chicken breast, it has more fat and sodium than a Big Mac. Since the chicken tastes so good (and after all, chicken is the "healthy choice"), you eat more of it than you normally would.

If I could state this so boldly, this is our problem: As Americans, we have been unknowingly manipulated into eliminating traditional diets meant for *satisfying* hunger and prodded into adopting high-caloric diets designed to *stimulate* our hunger.[4] And, because we are the richest nation in the history of the earth, we have unprecedented access to sugars, salt and fats!

It is easy to complain about the restaurant industry, but we addict ourselves to this cycle as well. We buy cheap junk foods because they're ready to eat or easy to prepare; and even though our bodies are telling us that we need good nutrition, we try to fool our bellies by feeding them sweets, fats and salt. This produces a "full" feeling temporarily, but soon our brains figure out that we still don't have the nutrition we need. When our brains remind us that we need nutrition, we fool them again by feeding our bellies more junk. The cycle goes on and on until we wake up 50 pounds overweight. Rick Ball was caught in this cycle until he decided he had had enough. He drastically reduced his consumption of sweets, fats and salt, and more than three years after giving his testimony in church, Rick continues to keep off the weight. "It still gives me a great feeling in the morning to get up and put on size 34 pants," says Rick. "We now have a granddaughter who was born in 2009, and I can keep up with her—I wouldn't have been able to do that before."

Eating Like Teenagers

Elizabeth Bailey also had to get tired of her condition before she did something about it. Having been a member of her high school track team, she fell prey to the habit that afflicts millions of people: eating the same way as adults that they did as teens. We often forget that the high level of activity in high school—when many of us are playing sports, running around town, shoveling snow or learning karate moves—helps burn up calories that don't disappear once we are sitting behind a desk.

In addition, Elizabeth's background worked against her. She describes her mother as a perpetually skinny woman who could eat everything in sight and never gain an ounce. Her father weighed in at around 300 pounds, reflecting his family's genetics—his parents were also overweight, and one of his sisters constantly fought a losing battle with yo-yo dieting. To make matters worse, when Elizabeth came into adulthood, she had not learned to cook, so she turned to cheap convenience foods at Marshall University.

"I was five-foot-seven and 115 pounds when I started college and just packed it on so slowly I didn't even realize I was doing it," she recalls. "That continued for 10 years, until I got up to around 210 or 215. I started getting really depressed about it. I lay on the couch and cried and said, 'What am I going to do?' My husband said, 'Get up and do something. Don't just lie there and cry.'"

Fortunately, Elizabeth found a way to reduce her excessive food intake. Not everyone does. Many get tripped up by the culture at home and a lack of cooperation from family, co-workers and friends. In an ideal world, those closest to us would support our efforts to improve our health. However, many people don't want to change, and they frown on anyone who upsets the status quo. Family members may resist and try to persuade you to return to old habits. Friends may make snide remarks about your eating, even when you never say a word. Some may shun you, since they feel judged by your discernment about what you put on your plate. You may be as loving and caring as ever, but they can't stand to see you getting slimmer while they continue to huff and puff around town.

If you let it, this will get to you. Too many people allow a lack of cooperation to become an excuse for their own lack of discipline. I've heard all kinds of complaints: "My kids won't let me exercise . . . my husband won't support me . . . nobody in my house likes that kind of food . . . what difference does it make? Aren't we going to heaven regardless of what we weigh?" I liken this to someone who decides to stop drinking because of alcohol's adverse affects. No sooner does a guy tell his friends he's gone sober than his buddies stop coming around and no longer want to socialize with him.

What's important to remember is that, just as those who stop drinking often report feeling better than ever, those who stop stuffing themselves feel happier, healthier, more vibrant, and more positive about life. I have seen this among successful participants in our church's Big Losers groups. They look better, have more energy, and are more pleased with themselves. They have a bounce in their step. I see a definite impact on their marriages. Because they aren't constantly tired, they are better able to care for their families. They even smile more often.

Eventually, Elizabeth succeeded and became one of these happy people. However, it took a long time to get tired of the feelings that came from looking at a picture of herself when she weighed over 200 pounds. It didn't help matters when her husband was deployed to Iraq with the Army Reserves. Although Elizabeth completed studies for her master's degree in reading education that year, she didn't want to spend off-campus hours alone. That led to frequent meals out with other military wives. This habit added to her weight problem, but spending time with those who understood her loneliness made her feel better.

The emotional high didn't last long. By the time her husband returned from Iraq, she felt terrible: "I just lay around all the time. I got so depressed I thought I had mononucleosis. When I was overweight, I would make believe I had hypoglycemia, and if I didn't eat I would get sick. On the one hand, I was confident enough to get my master's degree, but on the other hand, I was pitiful. I could put up a good front, though. Nobody knew how bad I felt inside. I tell people, 'Don't fool yourself. Anybody who is overweight doesn't like it; they hate it.'"

The Spiritual Solution

Elizabeth started on the journey toward better health in January 2006. By then, she had lost the 35 pounds she put on during pregnancy prior to the birth of her first son the year before. That still left her 100 pounds above her freshman weight. Through a weight loss workshop at our church, Elizabeth discovered that her battle with weight was spiritual in nature. She saw that she could only win with God's help.

She learned that her body was like a baby's, crying out for nourishment whenever hunger pangs hit. But instead of eating until she was full—or going over the line until her belly felt stretched out of shape—she learned to eat for contentment. Instead of conforming to society's dictates that she had to have three meals a day at certain hours, Elizabeth started eating only when necessary. That might mean lunch at 2 o'clock in the afternoon and dinner at 10 o'clock, or no dinner at all. When she felt impulses to eat, she read the Bible instead, and those feelings would pass.

"You hunger for the Word of God and hunger for His presence," she says. "You live on every word from the mouth of God. I learned that food wouldn't sustain me in the first place; it was God. I also learned that God expects me to obey Him. It was about being obedient and doing what He wants me to do. Eating whenever we want to eat is disobedient. It's like food becomes an idol. A lot of this is very abstract and spiritual. There was no formula. I just ate less, and I listened and paid attention to what God said."

Elizabeth drew so close to God that He became her primary support group. Each week, a pound or two drifted away—and after 10 months, she had lost more than 75 pounds. She expected potluck dinners at our church to be a difficult challenge, since they would offer some of the tempting treats that had defeated her in the past. However, because she wasn't following a traditional schedule, she often wasn't hungry when she came. So, she made sure her children had something to eat and then grabbed a glass of water or tea before chatting with friends.

To this day, for motivation, Elizabeth carries around a "before" photo of herself, taken when she started the weight loss workshop. Not only does it remind her of where she has been, but it also persuades those who don't think she can understand their struggles to open up and reveal their frustrations. Today, Elizabeth overflows with gratitude for God's help and the encouragement her husband, Dan, provided along the way. A longtime athlete and avid long-distance runner, Dan suggested she return to running. As the weight dropped off and she felt much lighter on her feet, Elizabeth took his advice. She ran her first race in years in the fall of 2006 and has been going ever since. In the fall of 2010, she completed a 10-miler in Washington, DC—and two weeks later, she completed her first half-marathon in Huntington.

"It helps me keep focused, I have time to talk to God, and it's a great stress reliever," Elizabeth says of her running routine. "I like to do it. I don't worry about time. My husband is really good; he ran the whole marathon in 3 hours and 12 minutes. When I ran the half-marathon, it took me 2 hours and 40 minutes. But, he's always encouraged me to do this stuff. He helped me with training and motivation. He went around the day of the half-marathon and told everyone how proud he was of me."

The week after starting his new routine, Rick Ball also recognized the divine help he had received. Noticing how much better he felt in just 10 days, he got on the scale for the first time and saw that he had already lost seven pounds. That prompted him to say, "Thank You, God!"—which made him realize he had left God out of the equation, never giving Him a thought when he started. "From that point on," Rick says, "I asked Him every day for His help—to help me watch what I ate and help me get healthy. I told Him, 'I want You to be in control. I need Your guidance and help to do this.'"

Keeping our focus on God instead of people is one secret to developing the perseverance to follow a healthy lifestyle. We aren't in this to please others or earn their praise, but to follow God's direction. As Paul puts it, "Whatever you do, work at it with all your heart, as working for the Lord, not for men, since you know that you will receive an inheritance from the Lord as a reward. It is the Lord Christ you are serving" (Col. 3:23-24). Says Rick, "If I think God's pleased with what I'm doing, I don't feel I owe anybody else anything. That's all I'm concerned with."

A New Lifestyle

As Rick's and Elizabeth's experiences show, even with God's help, you must adopt a new lifestyle and stick with it if you hope to see lasting change. This principle was illustrated clearly in our Big Losers program. The year it started, for the first two months nearly every person lost weight. However, those who said, "I'll try this for a few months and then go back to eating the way I want" inevitably failed. By contrast, participants who established and maintained new habits kept the weight off. Unless you make up your mind that this way of eating will last for the rest of your life, you will return to the "good old days." Speaking as one who used to lug around a few extra pounds, I can tell you that those days weren't so good.

Once you lose those pounds, however, I believe you won't want to go back. One way God keeps us moving forward is by providing encouragement from those around us. Elizabeth's and Rick's spouses were keys to their success. However, if you can't find support at home, develop it within the community or at church. Ask your pastor or a staff member about the possibility of developing a support network through a Sunday School class or special interest group. If none of that works, try a health club. People who work out at the YMCA or a gymnasium are more likely to be sympathetic to your desire to shed weight and shape up.

No matter where you find support, exercise is a necessary element of healthy living. The key is finding a workout you enjoy. Personally, I like swimming. For my wife, it's running. Others will hit the weight room. Some favor the group dynamics of an aerobics or Zumba class. No matter what you choose, at first it won't be much fun. Pushing yourself is a challenge until your body gets accustomed to the activity. You will get tired and possibly discouraged. Exercise takes planning, too, which adds a mental dimension to the discipline required. For example, I always had to think about the demands of my schedule for the week. If I knew I could only swim twice, I would do between a half-mile and a mile per session. If I knew I could swim four times, I might only swim between a quarter-mile and a half-mile per outing.

In addition to exercising, you must find healthy foods that are enjoyable. Nobody will stick with a constant routine of Brussels sprouts, carrot sticks and no-fat cheese (which one friend of mine insists is beyond redemption). My wife helped me adapt to healthier dinners. Jamie Oliver gave me some good recipes (which I have provided in the back of this book). For breakfast, I began blending fruit with protein shakes full of fiber and other nutrients. Protein and fiber helped fill me up without precipitating the sugar lows that came from eating too many carbohydrates. It took time for my stomach to get used to a liquid breakfast, but it works to this day.

We also had to adjust our outlook about feeling full. In the past, when I went to a restaurant, I thought, *If I'm going to spend $20 or more on an entrée, I want to leave here feeling full. I want to get my money's worth.* That is an American mindset that we need to leave on the scrapheap of history. Why? Because our stomachs expand as we feed them. If you get used to eating until you're full whenever you eat, each time you will have to eat more to achieve the same feeling. Eating to the point of fullness means eating too much. As Elizabeth learned, the better practice is to eat to the point of contentment. It is the scriptural principle of moderation, expressed by Paul in his letter to the Philippians: "I know what it is to be in need, and I know what it is to have plenty. I have learned the secret of being content in any and every situation, whether well fed or hungry, whether living in plenty or in want" (Phil. 4:12).

As you adapt to a new lifestyle, you may find it helpful to fix your eyes on the possibilities associated with weighing less. At his high mark in college, Brett Ballengee weighed nearly 300 pounds. As a result, he hesitated to volunteer to help with the teens' or younger children's activities at our church. He figured the only thing he would be good for was picking up a few stray balls or taking attendance. His church involvement consisted primarily of coming to Sunday morning services. That was a tragedy, especially in light of his degree in elementary education.

Even though he dropped about 10 pounds after graduation, Brett still got winded easily and felt terrible about himself. He didn't like making excuses about the extra pounds he carried on his six-foot, four-inch frame or hearing others excuse it with remarks like, "You're just a big guy." Thanks to his involvement in our first Big Losers group, Brett dropped more than 40 pounds and started showing a lot more energy. Soon thereafter, the youth pastor approached him and said, "I think you'd be really great to work with the high school kids." The same day, the children's director asked if he would be willing to run the games for elementary-age kids at our Wednesday night Awana program.

"Before, I was not able to serve and worship God with my body," Brett says. "I realized I could not serve in ways I was called to serve. I knew I wanted to work with kids. You don't get a degree in elementary education for the fun of it. You do it because you want to work with kids. The key thing for me was honoring and serving God with all my mind, soul and body, through being an active participant in the things I was asked to do. Putting my efforts and energy into focusing on what God had called me to do (lose weight), being obedient in that, and then God presenting an opportunity to serve—that was an encouragement. That was like God saying, 'You've been faithful and have followed what I called you to do, now here's an opportunity.'"

There is no guarantee that you will see such dramatic results as quickly as Brett did. However, when you change the way you're eating, you will see a new you emerging from behind the thick walls that are no doubt frustrating you and hiding your potential. It won't be easy, but it will be worth it. That much I know, from my own experience and from observing those around me who have taken this step towards a better life. As you shape up, remember the value of home-cooked meals. I will talk more about them as we step into the ring for Round 6.

Questions for Discussion

1. What do you think of the teens' diminished enthusiasm for Valerie's talk when she told them to stop drinking soda pop? In what ways are you like them?
2. Changing our lifestyles is not easy. Have you reached the point where the pain of an unhealthy lifestyle is greater than the pain of change? Why or why not? If not, what will it take for you to say, "That's enough!"?
3. Whose testimony did you identify with the most: Rick's, Elizabeth's or Brett's? What specific aspects of their lifestyle changes could help you in your journey?
4. How has our "sugar, fat and salt" culture most affected you? Which combination is your greatest weakness?
5. Following Daniel's biblical plan for change, how have YOU made up your mind to be different? Write down your specific, measurable goals for individual change. Be sure to have realistic timelines/deadlines by which these goals will be achieved.
6. Who will be your support group in your effort to improve your health? What else would motivate you? Be sure to include recruitment of these individuals in your overall plan for change.

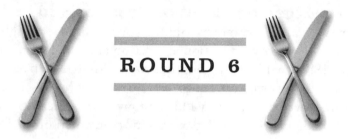

ROUND 6

There's No Place Like Home

Success in the restaurant business revolves around three crucial factors: location, location and location. In the same way, when it comes to winning your family's food fight, there are three keys to victory: education, education and education. Looking back, I can see that while raising our first two children, I didn't really care to learn about food or where it came from. Dee was more conscious of this issue, but whenever she was away I liked to give the kids candy and junk food. That made me the "cool" parent. However, when our third child reached school age, it quickly became obvious that certain foods caused him learning problems. That forced me to take nutritional education seriously. Suddenly I found myself lecturing his teachers on what he could and could not eat.

As I mentioned in the previous round, restaurants tap into our primal needs by injecting foods with all the sugar, fat and salt our taste buds can stand. It's no accident that the increase in our national obesity problems paralleled a rise in fat and oil consumption. Over a three-decade span starting in 1976, Americans' use of fats and oils increased 63 percent.[1] All this sugar, fat and salt not only put weight on us and our children, but also conditioned our kids to avoid healthy fruits and vegetables. In essence, we have hooked them on food that will lead them to an early grave. Who knew?

Honestly, haven't we all given something to our children thinking it wasn't so bad, only to find out later that we had contributed to the nutritional delinquency of a minor? After baseball practice, I used to buy our son a 20-ounce soda. Even when I noticed that it contained 58 grams of sugar, I thought, "What's the big deal?" (What in the world is a gram of sugar, anyway?) That was the problem. I hadn't educated myself on nutrition. Is 17 grams of fat a lot or a little? (Way too much, actually.) Many times I bought my children sugar-laden "juice drinks" or chicken sandwiches, thinking these were healthy options. I had no idea there was about a third of a cup of sugar in the average soda container or a Big Mac's equivalent of fat in a chicken sandwich. Why? Because I didn't know anything about how these are measured in foods.

Generally, 50 grams of sugar equals about a quarter-cup of the white stuff. Would you allow your child to go into the sugar jar, take out a spoon and straight-up eat a half-cup? Most parents wouldn't even consider that option, but what is the difference between that and a biggie-sized Mountain Dew (other than the fact that straight sugar isn't also loaded with caffeine)?

My knowledge of fast food was not much better. Even though Americans eat out an average of four to five times a week—and one-third of our children eat fast food *every single day*—most parents have no idea how much we overload kids with unneeded calories.[2] Until I woke up, I was guilty of this. While the average eight-year-old needs around 1,200 to 1,500 calories a day, the typical McDonald's "value meal" contains around 1,200 calories.[3] Gulp! Eating at sit-down restaurants can be just as bad or worse. The Center for Science in the Public Interest reports that it is common for appetizers alone to contain 2,000 calories (a full day's allotment for an average *adult*), with the main course offering another 2,000 calories. The average dessert checks in at 1,700 calories.[4]

The point is not to simply avoid fast-food outlets or restaurants. This isn't about behavior modification or piling more chores on our children so they can get plenty of exercise. Passing down healthy lifestyle habits ought to be every bit as important as passing on our faith. In fact, as I have discussed many times before, taking care of our bodies *is* a part of our faith.

Setting an Example

Eating the right foods and controlling portion sizes set a good example for our children. So does setting the tone for the way we live. Let's face it, when busy working parents have to get one child to ballet by 4 PM and another one to basketball at 4:30, it doesn't feel like they have much of a choice when it comes to good nutrition. Therein lies the problem: Too many American families are on the run.

I see this constantly as a parent, a coach and a pastor. Kids barely get home from school before it is time to dash out the door. By the time harried parents get all the kids picked up from lessons and practices, it's six or seven o'clock, and they have no idea what to fix for dinner. So what do they do? Hit the drive-thru window or call the pizza delivery boy. Fat and salt are on their way—a sugar-filled drink will save the day!

Pediatrician Amanda Workman sees around 3,500 patients annually at her Huntington office. She is constantly taken aback by the junk food her patients tote into the exam room. "It's amazing how much food they'll bring," she says. "We're right there in the office, and they're feeding the kids sugary snacks or pop. A lot of times you'll see a parent putting pop in a one-year-old's sippy cup. Sometimes it is other things that parents don't realize are unhealthy, like sugary fruit juice. They think, *That's from a fruit so it must be healthy*. Instead, it's full of sugar and empty calories."

When Dr. Workman points parents in the right direction, the mantra she often hears is, "But my kid won't eat that." Duh! Of course they won't eat healthy foods if we keep reinforcing their addictions to sugar, fat and salt. My guess is, if I gave my kids cigarettes and beer four days a week, they would probably balk at the idea of going back to the healthier option of chips and pop!

Part of winning the food fight is dictating nutritional choices. I cannot tell you how disheartening it is to see parents ruled by their children. Why do we get so stressed out because an eight-year-old is upset with us? Dee and I rarely force our kids to eat foods they don't like, and we try to be considerate of their preferences when planning our family menu; however, if they don't eat what Dee makes, we say, "You must not be *that* hungry." And that's it. Sometimes Dee feels sorry for them, but I'm not going to let them turn my wife (or me) into a short-order cook. Their dinner is on the table. If they are hungry, they can eat it.

When we weaned our children off salty foods, they didn't have much appetite for other things, and complaints abounded. We had to institute the old rule: "If you don't have something nice to say, don't say anything at all." That meant some quiet nights at the dinner table, but they got over it. Today, while they don't all love broccoli, they do eat *much* better. Lifestyle changes do not happen overnight, but they will happen if we're willing to make the effort over the long term."

I don't know about where you live, but around here, too many parents give their children whatever they want. Kids go to bed when they want, eat what they want, and watch whatever TV shows they want. Mom and Dad don't say much about it. (This is probably why the CDC says West Virginians are the worst when it comes to the amount of sleep they get—and naturally, this kind of indulgence spills over into our children's education as well.) In such an environment, it is no wonder that pediatricians like Dr. Workman face enormous challenges. More than half of her patients are overweight, and many are obese. She increasingly orders lab tests to check cholesterol and diabetes markers, regularly reviews body mass index readings, and finds herself referring children to a dietician.

"These problems are starting at a younger age all the time," Dr. Workman says. "With a handful of my patients, by the time they're reaching adulthood, they're already at a very scary health state. They're suffering from obesity-related health issues like high blood pressure, or they already have fatty liver disease. Or they have diabetes—not what used to be called juvenile or Type I, but Type II—at 18 or a little younger. It's just sad to see them in a state like that when they're just starting to be on their own—to have a life—and they're so large they can't move around."

Family Disintegration

This book is not just about food. Winning the food fight is just as much about understanding the underlying causes of our nutritional malevolence. Yes, a big problem is a lack of parental education and discipline. But perhaps there is even a greater cause for the problems we face as families. Our nation's love affair with fast food is one manifestation of a super-packed, fast-paced lifestyle that contributes to overall family disintegration.

I did the bulk of my Ph.D. studies on the causes of family breakdown. I can tell you unequivocally that it isn't healthy for families when Mom or Dad leaves work early, picks up a child at 3:30 or 4:00 PM, and whips through the drive-up window before rushing off to an evening practice. Our schedules are so tight that a full 20 percent of meals are now consumed in cars. (Not too great for the digestive process.) Just as bad, by the time our kids get home from practice, clean up and finish homework, there is hardly any time to build relationships and strengthen family ties. I believe with all my heart that God gave us food not only for sustenance, but also to slow us down so we could spend time with one another.

You may say, "Now, come on. Is it really *that* important for us to eat together around the dinner table?" Tons of research says, "Yes!" Various medical studies demonstrate the following benefits:

- *Healthier youth development.* Family "connectedness"—feelings of love, warmth and caring—has been consistently related to this. Doctors say that regularly sharing meals together is a method for developing and maintaining strong parent-child bonds.

• *Better nutrition.* Teens who dine with their families consume more fruits, vegetables and essential nutrients—and less junk food.

• *Better eating habits.* Families that make eating together a priority, provide rules and structure at mealtimes, and maintain an enjoyable atmosphere are *less* likely to see children engage in unhealthy eating and dietary behaviors. Children in these families also have reduced risk of eating disorders.

• *Preventing unhealthy behaviors.* You've probably heard the expression, "The family that prays together stays together." Well, I would amend it to: "The family that prays together and eats together stays together." Families who eat together have a much, much lower risk of divorce. In addition, connections formed around the dinner table are cited as reducing risks for children when it comes to emotional distress, substance abuse, involvement in violence, weight issues and early sexual behavior. Eating together also reduces the odds for use of cigarettes, alcohol and marijuana; problems with grades; and depression.[5]

When compared to teens who rarely have family dinners, those who have them five or more times a week are 42 percent less likely to drink alcohol, 59 percent less likely to smoke cigarettes, and 66 percent less likely to try marijuana. They are more than 300 percent less likely to abuse prescription drugs or an illegal drug other than marijuana, and less likely to be depressed. Teenage girls are less likely to use diet pills, laxatives or other extreme measures to control their weight. They are also 40 percent more likely to get As and Bs in school.[6] Says Marisa Weiss, M.D., president and founder of BreastCancer.org, "One of the most healthful medicines against breast cancer is family dinners. It is the single most potent way to improve your nutrition, manage your weight, feel support, find love, have fun, and create a family legacy of healthy eating."[7]

• *Additional benefits.* Other advantages to eating with your family include improved communication with your children, reduced stress and tension in the home, your children's friends being less likely to abuse prescription drugs, and increased likelihood that

your children will be willing to tell you about a serious problem.[8]
Children who have family dinners five or more nights a week
have greater language skills, expanded vocabulary, and articulate
their thoughts and feelings better.

"The practice of shared family mealtimes is a densely packed event
that bodes for either favorable or suboptimal child development," say Barbara H. Fiese and Marlene Schwartz, the authors of the report "Reclaiming the Family Table." "Shared family mealtimes have been associated with
such diverse outcomes as academic achievement, language development,
physical health, and reduced risk for substance abuse. . . . Shared mealtimes are an immensely symbolic event, not only for specific families, but
as a barometer of community health. . . . While only lasting twenty minutes
on average, family mealtimes are embedded in a social, cultural and economic context."[9]

On the other side of the coin, neglecting family time causes serious
problems. I have literally seen some families break up as a result of this
lack of bonding. For a while after I left home, my parents were separated.
I attribute that partially to their having run me around to so many practices, ballgames and other activities that we rarely had dinner or other time
together as a family. So, when I graduated, they discovered that they had
forged little common identity. Likewise, I have seen families stop coming
to church because they are so worn out from their frenzied pace. My question is: Why? I am sure that deep down most parents don't like living such
a harried lifestyle. Why do they remain slaves to the rat race?

This is the time when we have to do a reality check and evaluate
whether our children's potential will really be limited if we don't follow
the numb-minded herd. If we want our children to succeed at the most
important things—like being good spouses and loving parents when they
grow up—then we need to engage in such old-fashioned habits as setting
limits and forming priorities. After all, Abraham Lincoln didn't play Little League, George Washington couldn't play *Canon in D*, and Susan B. An-
thony never led cheers for her high school team. Great leaders don't develop
fortitude by following the crowd. Yes, we need to develop various skills in
our children, but we should never do this at the expense of God's most
important institution: the family.

Long ago, my wife and I decided we wouldn't force (or allow) our children to participate in things that required many multiple-night practices.

We limit each child to two outside activities, such as sports and music lessons. With our kids already in or nearing their teens, this has been a key to maintaining our habit of eating dinner together at home at least three or four nights a week (plus we eat a home-cooked dinner together at church on Wednesdays).

Parents often come to me as a pastor and say that their child is stressed out and isn't responding well to discipline at home or at school. I usually ask them about their family dinner time, and they typically respond that they don't have a normal schedule so they can't have a family dinner. According to child development specialist Dr. Harvey Karp, meals are important, even to the youngest children. "Having predictable routine for toddlers lowers stress, increases their confidence, and makes them feel smarter, because they know what to expect. Routines like dinner are an island of calm in a world of change. They are predictable and anchoring."[10]

Eating Through a Window

As a nation, if our families are going to win the food fight, eating on the run must become a thing of the past. Yes, the average child eats fast food often, but who wants their child to be average? I have read a number of books on eating out, searched multiple research articles, and asked several physicians and nutritionists how often it is "okay" to eat fast food. Their answers ranged from "never" to "two or three times a month." Did you catch that? Not one authoritative source recommended eating fast food even weekly. Most said it was never good, but sometimes life might demand it. If you want a healthy family, prepare healthy meals at home.

Once you have made that decision, it is time to develop a plan. Set a standard. Decide to have dinner around the table (not in the family room in front of a TV) several nights a week. Be realistic. If you have teens with packed schedules, you may have to start with one night a week. Once a week is better than never, and one night could turn into two or three. Time with family should dictate participation in outside activities. The way most people operate, activities dictate their time together as a family.

When it comes to family dinners, I credit Dee with making them a priority, particularly during my days as a youth pastor. I sure hope you don't think I've been too preachy, because I assure you that in this area,

I was the chief of sinners. Back when I worked with teens, I attended ballgames, band concerts, cheerleading competitions and youth group events almost every night. With 100 teenagers in our youth group, plus 300 more who connected through school clubs or athletics, I felt like I was the father of 400 children. My biological children were toddlers then, and I didn't value family time as much as my wife did. I'm thankful she insisted I come home for dinner before heading out the door again.

Another of Dee's major contributions has been wisely managing our household expenses. I realize that some households necessitate two full-time incomes, but for more than 10 years, we raised three children on a salary that averaged less than $30,000 a year. It can be done. But I am convinced that it *could not* have been done if we had eaten out four nights a week and incurred the expenses of multiple extracurricular activities.

Dee's domestic management skills include planning our dinner schedule. She used to follow a more precise plan in buying groceries for the week. Now she just makes sure we have enough food in the house so she can adjust as needed. If she knows it will be a hectic day, in the morning she puts something in the Crockpot to simplify dinner preparations.

"Sometimes we'll have lasagna on Sunday, and I'll just program the oven before church in the morning and when we get home it's ready," she says. "I think that's the biggest thing—just planning so you know you have food in the house and you know what you can have for dinner that night. You also have to factor in schedules and how much time you will have to prepare the meal. One night we might go casual and eat a bowl of cereal or something, but we still have time together."

Dee picked up a great idea from Laurie David's *The Family Dinner*, which suggests having theme nights, such as Taco Tuesday or Breakfast Dinner Thursday. She finds it one of the best books she has read on encouraging family dinner times. And, as I mentioned earlier, having a plan helps stimulate creativity. Once the theme is set, Dee searches for healthy alternatives within that framework. I always look forward to what she and the kids will come up with when I come home in the evening.

By contrast, when I was a teen, our primary methods for eating looked more like a typical, rushed family. Most of our dinners happened in one of these ways: (1) Mom made something, set it on the counter, and I swooped through, took some food and sat in front of the TV; (2) I grabbed something out of the refrigerator, whether leftovers, a bowl of cereal or frozen pizza; or most often (3) we headed for the nearest fast-food outlet.

Please hear what I am about to share. I love my parents dearly, and later in this book I have a lot of good things to say about them. They did the best they knew how. But if I am going to be honest, I have to say that the family I grew up in is nothing like the family I have now. My parents centered their lives around raising me. While it seemed good then, I did not enter marriage with a decent understanding of what it meant to be a good husband or a spiritual leader to my children.

I thank God that I married a woman who, even at the tender age of 20, had a solid understanding of what she wanted her family to look like. Dee had good examples from her own family and built on that foundation through extensive reading. She took seriously articles about how making conversation around the dinner table the norm created a close-knit family—and how if natural conversation was the pattern children followed, as they entered their teen years it would create open communication. With two children in their teens and the third almost there, I can see how making our family a priority has paid off. Sure, our children are spreading their wings (it's a normal part of growing up), but our relationships are in great shape. In large part, that is because of family dinners.

The good news is, once kids get the feel for family-style dinners, they tend to like them. Each summer, I speak at a high school camp in the mountains of central West Virginia. Camp Cowen is a throwback of sorts. When it's time to eat, kids don't go through a cafeteria line. Instead, they sit around 10-person tables and share family-style meals. Camp Director Rob Ely once considered going to a faster, more efficient system, but after observing the quality of conversation around the dinner tables, he decided against it. "We've had a lot of kids tell us this is the only time of the year when they sit down and talk during a meal," Rob says. "It's amazing the relationships that are developed around food. Conversations take place in our dining halls that probably never would occur if kids just came in, ate their food, and went right back out the door."

I conducted a little poll among some former campers, asking if they would have preferred a cafeteria-style line—if that meant they would have more free time after meals. Not one student liked the idea. "My favorite memories of camp are sitting in the dining hall and talking with my counselors," one said. "Most of the day was busy with activities, but every time we ate, I had a chance to have some quality conversations that changed my life." My prayer is that someday your children will say the same thing about your family dinners.

Making the Change

As you strive to transition toward home-cooked, healthy meals, you may want to take a lesson from Heather Lucas, coordinator of the Mothers of Preschoolers (MOPS) program at our church and mother of four children. Despite busy schedules, the Lucases take steps to ensure that they eat healthily. Like Dee, Heather makes regular use of her Crockpot—something that can become a lifestyle habit. Freezer cooking is another strategy: Heather prepares several meals, freezes them, and cooks them later. She is also fond of making a picnic lunch or taking along crackers, peanut butter and fresh fruit to the ball field on Saturdays. Not only does that enable the Lucases to avoid fast food, but it also offers a family-style dinner in the park.

One does not have to be a stay-at-home mother to sit down with her family for dinner. Dr. Workman married a single father in the spring of 2009. Since then, she and her husband have been sticklers for shared family meals, despite her medical practice and his busy schedule as a contractor. She admits it has taken quite an adjustment to make sure they have the right food on hand to make healthy meals, but she says it is worth the effort. Their meal challenges include navigating an 11-year age difference between the oldest and youngest of their three kids.

"It's big," she says of family dinners that are often cooked by her husband. "It gives us time to interact with the kids by sitting down face to face and talking about our day or something we have planned. Especially with the differences in ages in our house, everyone's doing something different. We might be reading a book, playing on the computer, or running off to this activity. Dinner gives us the time where we have each other's attention and we're sharing something on our minds—dreams, plans or whatever it is. It opens the door to conversation."

Overcoming Resistance

When it comes to getting your children to eat healthier foods, sometimes you have to be a little creative. On his mini-series, Jamie Oliver recommended putting fresh vegetables in tomato sauce and other dishes, something Heather Lucas has done for years. She uses carrots in numerous dishes, since they tend to take on the flavor of whatever they are cooked with. Dee suggests experimenting with different vegetables and other dishes, as well as trying raw veggies. Since most vegetables are healthier raw, she often will serve a spinach salad instead of cooking and creaming it. She also substitutes whole grain pasta for white and has dropped white bread for whole wheat.

It is important to sample new foods regularly, since it takes repeated "tastes" to appreciate a new flavor. One recommendation is to keep trying different things gradually and remember that tastes change. More than once we've told our kids, "Just because you didn't like it last year doesn't mean you won't like it this year."

Setting the Standard

Healthy eating involves more than family dinners and wise meal planning. As I mentioned earlier, parents must embrace their #1 duty as role models and set a good example. That responsibility inspired Heather Lucas to shed 50 pounds after the birth of her fourth child in 2006. She had to develop discipline after carrying around extra weight for six years, ever since the birth of her second child. After she and Larry decided their family was complete, Heather looked inward and decided she was tired of obesity.

"I felt like it was bad for my health, and it wasn't good for the kids either," she says. "I knew that I needed to be active so I could take them to the pool or the amusement park. I wanted to be an active mom who played around with them, had fun, and wasn't tired all the time. I wanted to be able to keep up. We got strict with healthier eating—eating more vegetables and fruits. It was about six months before I reached my goal. For the most part, my eating habits changed, and I haven't gone back."

Dr. Workman calls modeling by parents the key to solving childhood obesity, exhorting parents to eat healthy foods with their kids. Unfortunately, many parents would rather watch their kids get fat than change their own habits. "Rarely will I see two physically fit parents come in with a severely obese child," reports Dr. Workman. "The problem almost always continues generationally. I know genetics plays somewhat of a factor, but for the most part, if Mom and Dad learn how to discipline their own eating habits, they will pass that along to their children."

Let's Get Physical

Parents play a vital role in another key element of the food fight equation: exercise. Many kids become couch potatoes by observing those closest to them. Since her children are involved in sports, Heather doesn't have to prod them to run and play, but she still does her part by running. In the summer of 2010, she got involved in the "Couch-to-5K®" running plan.[11] That enabled her to run her first 5K race that October and participate in our church's second annual Thanksgiving 5K the following month.

In addition, Heather says mothers and fathers can reduce childhood obesity through scheduling activities that emphasize physical fitness. "You can do things as a family that don't revolve around food," Heather says. "I think it's important for bonding time and to get to know each other and spend time together. My husband pretty much coaches every sport our children play. Our whole family attends each other's events whenever possible. We are always there to support each other and cheer each other on."

At our house, we strive to stay active because we want our kids to grow up physically fit and teach our grandchildren this lifestyle. Dee is a runner; I like to swim and play sports. We regularly plan vacations around places where we can hike and take in the beauty of nature. Since we live on a hill, Dee often encourages our kids to go out and play games or just run up and down the hill.

"That is the big problem for kids," she says. "When we were kids, we were outside and running around all the time. I had a friend whose mother would lock the door when she left and tell her, 'Just stay outside.' I know we cannot do that today. Now, all kids are into video games. They aren't getting fresh air and running around and playing as much."

Much to Dee's chagrin, I like gaming systems too. My boys and I used to play games all afternoon, but thankfully Momma put a stop to that. Now they (or should I say "we") can play a half-hour in the evening and that's it. On the weekends, we can play during the day, but it's still only a half-hour. Although technology has put a damper on exercise, it does have an upside, particularly in the winter. When we bought a Nintendo Wii system, we purchased dance mats that the kids use for exercising with fitness games when it gets dark early or is too cold for outdoor activities.

Our other new love is geo-caching, which combines hiking and treasure hunting. The kids complain when we load them up for a treasure hunt, but as soon as we get close to the geo-cache, the competition is on. They race around the park, woods or ball fields to find the hidden treasure. Occasionally our oldest son will catch himself having too much fun and revert to "Joe Cool" teenager. That's all right. I know he's having a good time even if he doesn't want to admit it. Ten years from now, the memories my kids will share on holidays will revolve around our outdoor activities, not a video game.

Train Them Up

Helping your children develop good exercise habits has both immediate and long-term benefits, as kids who exercise are more likely to become adults who exercise. Heather Smith is a member of the Huntington Health Revolution (more about this group in Round 8) and oversees fitness programs at the Marshall University recreation center. She is shocked by how many students come to college overweight and out of shape. How bad is it? Of the hundreds of students who attend her various fitness sessions, at least 50 percent are overweight and another 25 percent are borderline. Often Heather has to scale back the exercises she planned because so many of her students have poor endurance.

This lack of fitness starts in childhood. Some kids in our area are in such bad condition that they've been ordered by their physicians to enlist personal trainers. While they could be running around at home to get the same exercise, a lot of parents are uneducated about how simple exercise can be. "A lot of [the parents] are overweight, so they're sending them to someone who can be a good example," Heather says. "Still, with a lot of these kids, fitness training is saving their lives. They're at risk of Type II diabetes because they're overweight and so unfit."

In the face of such factors, parents who really want their children to get healthy and fit will do something about it. Heather recommends:

1. Encouraging them to do something active outside of school. They don't have to jog several miles, but they must do something to stay active. This can include the whole family exercising, playing games, or doing house or yard work.

2. Recognizing the importance of *portion control*, including limiting what children consume. It's not just that our families are eating the wrong foods; they're also eating too much of them. On the rare occasion of eating out, we need to stop supersizing. (Children NEVER need a 20-ounce bottle of soda pop. Have you noticed that sodas that used to come in 12-ounce cans gradually inflated to 20-ounce bottles? This is overkill.)

3. Setting an example by eating healthy and exercising: "If parents take care of their own health, that's a huge factor. Over the years, there has been a gradual decline in physical activity

and family meals, and a gradual increase in eating processed foods. I think it's going to take gradual improvements to change that. It's a battle, but it's one we can take on."

As If Your Life Depended on It

I conclude this round with the story of Don and Faith Hartman, friends from Dallas. In 1996, they were overjoyed over the birth of their second child and first son, Brendan. He registered a perfect 10 on his APGAR score—an acronym that stands for appearance, pulse, grimace, activity and respiration. Everyone breathed a sigh of relief that mother and child were healthy. At this point, I'll let Faith take over:

"At his two-week check-up, the pediatrician felt our son's liver was a bit big and ordered some tests. The doctor followed his blood test with an urgent sonogram late in the day. He called us immediately with the results, saying he would book an 8 AM appointment for us the next morning. The urgency in his voice alarmed me. Although the pediatric gastroenterologist was booked for six months, he still worked us in. He explained it could be a virus, or bad food, or a rare, awful condition called 'biliary atresia,' where the liver is totally blocked."

Since this was before the Internet was so common, Don and Faith went to the medical library to educate themselves about biliary atresia and what it does to the body. The pictures of kids with malformed and misshapen faces were heartbreaking.

"We finally learned Brendan would need surgery," Don says. "The odds weren't good—a third of children die anyway, a third do well, and a third are 'wait and see.' While we were waiting through the five-hour surgery, God showed us in the Bible that almost everyone who asked Jesus for healing did so on their faces, so that's how we prayed. Ever since, we've done that as a family. We saw answers to that and other prayers—we identified 134 distinct miracles in Brendan's healing. One was the busy, godly surgeon who came to see us in the hospital. At that point, we weren't even sure if our son had biliary atresia, and we hadn't chosen this surgeon to operate. But it turned out he had learned the special bypass surgery and did the first of these operations in Dallas 25 years earlier.

"After surgery, Brendan was 'wait and see.' They said he would probably need a liver transplant, although they didn't know if that would be in 5, 10 or 20 years. While we had a wonderful, compassionate pediatric gastroenterologist, when we asked if there was anything we could do to help his chances with diet, the doctor said, 'No.' Like the old joke about the guy hanging off a cliff, we asked, 'Is there any other help up there?'"

Despite the discouraging response from Brendan's doctor, the Hartmans continued to research the topic—and then a friend gave them a tape of Dr. Joel Robbins explaining the medical reasons that fresh fruits and vegetables are so good for us. Don explains, "If he didn't also have a medical degree, I don't think I would have listened. In the end, we didn't have any other options. We learned that God has made the human body with a great ability to fight disease and heal itself with the right nutrition—along with clean air, water, sunshine and sleep."

Operating on faith, as well as reason, Don and Faith arranged their budget so they could switch Brendan's diet to 100 percent fresh or raw foods, including fresh fruit and vegetable juice. Obviously their child's health was a priority to them, and they took the steps necessary to ensure that all of their children had access to proper nutrition. The results were simply fantastic.

Over the next few months, Brendan steadily grew healthier, with his check-ups going from weekly to monthly. Then they faded to quarterly, and finally to annually. "Early on we were nervous—until Brendan started getting better and better, growing healthier at each stage," says Don. "He is a strapping teenager now and doing fine."

When it comes to good health, many people will protest that they just cannot afford gym memberships or proper foods. In the mid-1990s, most Americans didn't have 42-inch flat screen TVs or cell phones, or pay $50 a month for Internet services, but today most families have arranged their finances so they can afford these non-essentials. The same families that "cannot afford" to make healthy food and exercise choices come up with cash for expensive athletic shoes, practice jerseys and cheerleading uniforms. For the Hartmans, eating healthier meant a major financial adjustment, but their child's life literally depended on it.

The question is: What do you value? Do you value physical health more than a nicer car, an iPhone or gaming systems? We all make choices. As for me and my house, we have chosen our children's long-term health.

From healthy families come healthy churches. See what yours can do in Round 7.

Questions for Discussion

1. Why is education so important when it comes to your family's nutrition? What mistakes do most families make?
2. How often do you have dinner at home as a family? What could you do to increase the frequency? What benefits would more meals around the dinner table have for your family?
3. If you have teens involved in numerous activities, how could you prioritize your schedule to have more dinners together?
4. Are your children picky eaters? How did they get that way? What could you do to persuade them to make some changes?
5. What kind of exercise are your children getting? Are there activities you could do as a family?
6. What are three lessons we can learn from the Hartman family?

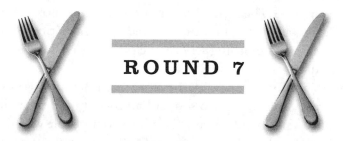

ROUND 7

Our Church Isn't Growing

(And We're Happy About It)

On a 2010 trip to the Philippines, Huntington pastor Chuck Lawrence saw a first-hand demonstration of the difference healthy eating makes. His experience emphasizes how Americans' embrace of rich foods is ruining their lives and sending millions to an early grave. The events I am about to describe took place in Cebu, on South Cabato, an island on the eastern edge of the nation. After Chuck preached at a church's morning service, the pastor offered to show him the countryside during an afternoon break.

As they headed up a mountain, the pastor said, "I want to show you the top; this is a really neat view." No sooner had they started their climb than the pastor made an offhand remark about the poor people who lived in the area. Indeed, as Chuck looked out, he saw half a dozen youngsters playing volleyball. Obviously lacking equipment, they were using a soccer ball, with a frayed rope stretched between a pair of crude, wobbly-looking sticks as the net. Behind them, some chickens wandered around the hillside, which brimmed with leafy green vegetables, corn, carrots and other plants. What stood out, though, were these young men's muscular physiques. Their arms and abs rippled with the kind of fit, toned muscles that Americans would shell out thousands of dollars to achieve. Gesturing toward the volleyball game, the robust pastor—though not obese, he definitely carried extra weight—remarked, "These are poorer kids in this area. It's really sad. They have to eat off this hill. That's because they're so poor."

"He didn't even realize what he was saying," Chuck says, smiling. "He was implying, 'They don't have a chance to go to the restaurants I do; they don't have a chance to eat all the great food I get to eat. Instead, they have to eat off the hill.' But they were in immaculate shape. I have never forgotten that. We would do ourselves a great favor if we would learn to eat off the hill."

Since 2002, Chuck has been persuading members of his church, Christ Temple, to follow a lifestyle that will enable them to boast the kind of physique that those "poor" Filipinos achieved by eating off the hill. This emphasis originated in the late 1990s, when a friend of Chuck's pointed out the overwhelming number of foods containing hydrogenated oils. These specially processed oils extend the shelf life of foods to formerly unheard-of spans. However, since our bodies can't easily process them, they cause us to pack on pounds. A couple of years after Chuck and his wife, Jamie, started making a conscious effort to avoid these oils, they looked so fit that church members asked what they were doing. That led to a sermon series Chuck titled "Fit for Purpose."

When members complained that they couldn't find the health foods Chuck talked about in his sermons, Jamie created a natural foods section at the church bookstore. Though since scaled back, it initially carried such items as natural sugar, whole-wheat flour, organic milk, organic peanut butter, and drinks that didn't use high-fructose corn syrup. Enough people asked about such alternatives while shopping that stores like Kroger's and Wal-Mart added health food sections—a first for this area. One Christ Temple member even helped design the section at a Kroger's in neighboring Ashland, Kentucky.

None of this happened overnight, which illustrates how improving health is a long-term effort. I'm not the least bit upset that Christ Temple started this emphasis long before our church joined the parade. In fact, I'm encouraged to see how God works in multiple ways to get His message across to His people. Thank God, folks at Christ Temple got the message and formulated plans for a fitness center on church grounds. Although it took eight years to complete the project, today the center is stocked with stationary bicycles, treadmills, elliptical machines, Stairmasters, weight machines and free-standing weights. To promote ongoing exercise, they offer sessions with a physical trainer for $10 an hour, one-third the area's going rate. Health center memberships include a discount card that can only be used at health-oriented restaurants.

A Core Belief

"What we've done is make it a core belief," Chuck says of the gradual expansion of "Fit for Purpose" into numerous areas of church life. "We're not trying to browbeat them; we're trying to encourage them and we do that consistently."

"For example, if we have a large dinner here, like we do at Christmastime, we will not put out margarine because of the hydrogenated oils in it," says Jamie, who has played a key role in spreading awareness of healthy living. "So even though we're not overtly teaching, we're teaching by example, by modeling behavior. We don't ever mention weight. It's not about weight. It's about health and your purpose in life. The weight loss is kind of a byproduct of living a healthy life."

"It's woven into everything we do," Chuck adds. "People around here are poorer than in other places. Even if they don't think about it, if they get an opportunity to eat, they want to eat as much as they can. It's kind of woven into their fabric. People tend to overeat because more food means a better meal."

Despite years of this emphasis, Chuck estimates only 25 percent of the 1,800 or so who attend Sunday services at Christ Temple have bought in to this message. Such relatively low success rates might sound discouraging, but they reflect our experience in our church as well. After I gave my first sermon on healthier living, close to 60 people signed up for our Big Loser competition—but fewer than half made it to the end. People look at such numbers in two ways. Some see a glass filled to half its capacity while others moan that it is half-empty. Some of our lay leaders get discouraged over the ones who fade away, but I get excited about those who persevere. If 60 people sign up, and only 30 complete their goals, that is still 30 more than we had in the first place. That's 30 more who know the blessing of achieving lofty goals and serving God more effectively.

Don't miss the importance of fitness in your future. America's ethic emphasizes early retirement, but God's purpose is for people to remain active and accomplish feats well into their senior years. Think of Noah building the ark, Abraham raising young Isaac, Moses leading the slaves out of Egypt, Daniel facing the lions, or Peter leading the Church in Rome—all done after age 60. Joshua and Caleb were warriors in their eighties! The idea is to stay healthy so you can serve the Lord for as long as possible.

"Everything you're going to do in your lifetime is going to be done in your physical body," Chuck says. "I know numerous people who are not able to do what they want to do because their physical body will not cooperate. I believe that when God gave them that body, He also gave them a purpose. That purpose was intended to be fulfilled in that body. If their physical body has been inundated by improper physical habits—everything from food to a sedentary lifestyle—that leads to not having the energy they need or the health to fulfill His purpose. Everyone needs to maximize what God has given to them, and the way to do that is through a healthy lifestyle."

Start Somewhere

After my introductory sermon on obesity, our church's entry into healthy living started with a single initiative: Big Losers. As I mentioned, the first class attracted 60 people. Participants were divided into three groups that met on different nights. Each group met weekly for exercise, accountability, exchanging ideas and prayer. They also weighed in once a month, and the team that lost the most weight won a prize. Were that the only thing we did, our emphasis would still have been a resounding success. You may wonder why I say that, when more than half of the people in the first group of classes faded away. Two reasons:

- Those who stuck with the program have reaped such rewards as losing weight, getting rid of medications and experiencing healthier lifestyles. In the first two years of Big Losers, members collectively lost a ton of weight.

- The weight loss effort sparked additional steps that created multi-faceted options for those who want to be better stewards of their bodies.

The Big Losers group features the kind of simple concept that any church or community group can implement. Meet weekly for an hour or two of instruction, devotional time and exercise, and do periodic weigh-ins. Don't wait until you can enlist enough "experts" before you get started. All you need is someone who cares enough to hold others accountable and live out healthy principles in his or her life.

Although neither has a degree in physical fitness or expertise in health, Elizabeth Bailey and her husband, Dan, have helped coach several groups. Elizabeth has a master's in education, but her current job is raising their children. Dan is a civil engineer. Others who have led groups work in such occupations as public information, office administration and children's programming.

"You just have to love people enough to care to help them get there," Elizabeth says. "A lot of times I didn't have to tell them, 'This is how you do it' and spell out the ABCs. I just told them about myself and helped encourage them. They knew what to do. They understood that they have to eat less and exercise more."

The Baileys follow the three-part concept I outlined in my sermon by addressing physical, educational and spiritual issues. While all three are important, it was the last area that provided the key to Elizabeth's weight loss—and is essential to all of us. Exercise alone won't provide the answer, nor will knowledge. When it comes to improving your health, the key is understanding who made you, who is in charge of your body, and whom you are to obey.

Because of her focus on the spiritual element of weight control, in her first class Elizabeth initially led the devotional sessions—finding inspiration for these discussions in her own daily Bible readings. She shared with the class her technique for dealing with hunger pangs. "When I felt hungry, I read the Bible."

Gradually, the Baileys turned all aspects of Big Losers into a participatory program. As group members gained confidence, they were invited to lead exercise sessions, educational studies on various food topics, and devotions. The more individual members took ownership of the program, the more success the group achieved.

"Do something—anything," Elizabeth says. "Have a walking club or an aerobics class. You can even use a video if you don't have someone who can be an instructor. Do something—anything—instead of just talking about it."

"You don't even need facilities," Dan says. "At first, we did many of the exercises in the church hallways. We ran up and down stairs and used soup cans as weights. With the initial class, we were in the middle of a construction project, and one night we used construction materials for exercise. We took bricks and built walls with them. You don't have to have a gym or a health club membership. You don't have to have a set of weights or fancy equipment or the right clothes . . . the bottom line is to do something."

You Go, Girl!

Nancy Carpenter is one of Big Losers' success stories. The mother of two grown children, she shed 75 pounds, along with her blood pressure medication. Her doctor had wanted to increase her dosage after her blood pressure reached 142 over 95, but by eating healthier she lowered it to 90 over 69. Today she is more outgoing, the result of a newfound confidence she previously lacked because she didn't think she could accomplish anything. Despite her struggles with self-worth, until I preached about obesity, Nancy didn't think she needed to lose weight, because others regularly commented on how healthy she looked.

"People didn't realize how heavy I was," she recalls. "I must have hidden it well. I had allowed myself to be driven by food and not what I needed to be doing. You don't realize what you're doing to yourself with food. I got lazy and contented, and it was easier to sit down and eat what I wanted without thinking about it. It just drifted on over the years, particularly when I took a new job in 2003. In my new job, I just sat day after day and ate out all the time—pizza, sandwiches, anything. In the past, I cleaned and did housekeeping, so I was always moving or going after the kids."

The classes' spiritual component helped open Nancy's eyes. Reflecting on her condition, Nancy realized that carrying around this much weight kept her from fulfilling God's intentions for her life. In addition to gaining insights from class devotions, every morning she visited an Internet weight loss site for inspiration. One primary lesson God taught her was that she had more strength than she thought. He showed her there was a healthier woman inside, just waiting to break out. All she had to do was cooperate.

The classes introduced accountability to Nancy's life; weighing in every other week kept her honest. Since groups competed in teams to see who could lose the most, she didn't want to let her teammates down. She didn't want to let me down as her pastor, either. Positive peer pressure entered into the picture as well. The group reinforced the goal of healthy living, counteracting our culture's embrace of all-you-can-eat buffets and ridicule of thin people. Now that she has lost so much weight, one old friend calls her anorexic and others label her skinny. Such comments just bring a smile to her face. Nancy is not only healthier but also more relaxed.

Losing weight initially at the rate of two pounds a week gave her the desire to keep going once the class ended. Her success has motivated her to mentor other women—including one struggling with diabetes—and encourage them to follow the road to good health. Her achievement includes keeping the weight off despite quitting cigarettes eight months after completing Big Losers. Just giving up nicotine after 35 years was a major accomplishment, symbolizing how gaining control of her eating transferred to other areas.

"It was something I had wanted to do for years," says Nancy, a dispatcher for the Kenova Police Department. "It was like a light bulb went off, and I was done. I've kept the weight off by doing 30 to 45 minutes every day on the treadmill in bad weather. In the summer, I'm out walking three miles a day. I'm just a lot happier now."

Big Losers helped Beth Smith see how much of an idol food had become. Though being her household's grocery shopper and cook made a certain amount of focusing on food necessary, Beth realized she devoted too much time to thinking about food and placed too high a premium on its pleasures. Her weight problem had started in 2000, after her mother died and she quit smoking. Beth lost 20 pounds on her own, and then the classes helped her shed 40 more. In the process, she lowered her cholesterol from 214 to 146. That helped her avoid the medication her doctor had suggested.

Beth also gained a new perspective.

"I learned to be content with everything God has given me," says Beth, who wants to lose another 20 pounds. "A lot of things God gives us are pleasing. Food is one of those things, but we need to use moderation. I like the verse, 'So whether you eat or drink or whatever you do, do it all for the glory of God' (1 Cor. 10:31). If I overeat, I can't follow some other commands He has given me, like serving Him and loving Him with all my mind, soul and strength."

Wherever you are in your personal journey, don't let guilt weigh you down. At first Beth felt like a failure for not taking care of her body, which she knew is a temple of God. She acknowledges that some guilt is good—we certainly don't want to feel good about ourselves after a gluttonous outbreak—but the classes showed her she could do something about her problems. The mutual support helped; she liked hearing how others overcame their struggles. Classmates also shared healthy meal alternatives, recipes and cooking tips. It comforted Beth to know that she wasn't alone in her struggles and that her success could encourage others.

"One of the keys was coming to the realization that overeating is wrong," Beth says. "A lot of people aren't aware of that. We know we're not supposed to be a drunk or abuse drugs, but when it comes to food, we don't talk about that much. Coming to that realization helped me more than anything else."

Exercise Enthusiast

A premier booster of Big Losers now lives in the Washington, DC, area. Although he only lived in West Virginia for two years while serving as an intern with the Veterans Administration, Kregg Parenti gained a lifelong benefit. In January 2009, he tipped the scales at 306 pounds. Dan Bailey invited Kregg to try a few Big Losers sessions. Kregg enjoyed the varied exercise routine, and soon he brought his entire family. By the end of 2010, Kregg had lost 66 pounds and had turned into an avid exercise enthusiast.

"This time it clicked," he says, acknowledging a past failed attempt to get healthier. "I recognized that I needed exercise to be a part of my life. I try to do something daily where I'll burn calories, even if it's only 300 or 400, and get my metabolic rate going. On the weekends, I burn 2,000 calories with combined running and walking. Big Losers helped me realize a couple of things. One was the value of a small group and being able to talk about frustrations, pray for one another, and have a night where we got together on a consistent basis. If I had been by myself, I wouldn't have done anything."

The second insight Kregg gained was a biblical perspective on health. He saw how coming together for accountability to weight loss and exercise goals mirrors the Christian life in general. Each of us needs others' input for moral support and insight. Not only does this strengthen us for life's often-difficult journey, but it also helps us refocus on what is important. Kregg transferred these principles to his new job by enrolling in an employee wellness program, which includes a lifestyle coach. During weekly calls, Kregg's coach asks if he is still meeting exercise and weight loss goals. "That helps," he says.

Like Elizabeth Bailey, Kregg carries before-and-after pictures to remind him of the bad old days. Because of his experience, he knows that a happy-go-lucky, jovial personality can mask what is going on inside. In his case, he was sick of looking like the Pillsbury Doughboy™ and lacking energy. Nor did he want his four children to grow up looking like him. "I got tired of looking the way I looked," Kregg says. "I didn't want this anymore. I didn't want my kids to struggle with food or exercise like I had. Now I feel more energetic and more alert.

"One thing my wife noticed is that before, when we went out to eat, she always wanted to sit in a booth, but I never did. I got tired of the table hitting me in the gut. Now it's not an issue. I also like being able to have enough energy to do what the kids want to do, like going on hikes instead of staying home and watching TV."

Big Losers inspired additional activities, such as our annual Thanksgiving 5K run. It also stimulated a year-round exercise program, thanks in part to Jamie Oliver's fund-raising boost that enabled us to complete our family life center. After finishing construction, in early 2010 we started walking groups and exercise classes. After joining one group, our music minister set a goal of walking 100 miles per month. I thought that was a bit ambitious, but he did it. As a result, he lost 20 percent of his body weight and now wears the same size jeans he wore in college. This shows the power of accountability in a group environment.

Teaching Mature Dogs New Tricks

When I first challenged our congregation to adopt healthier lifestyles, my biggest concern was how my exhortation would be received by some of our older members. I don't know why I was so concerned. These people have always treated me like a son. They love me, and they know that I love them.

But even in my wildest dreams, I never anticipated how much ownership our senior adults would take in this process. One of our most vibrant go-getters, Loretta Gallion, coordinates volunteers to open up our family life center each day. Dozens of retired folks exercise there daily, and Loretta has embraced the task of encouraging walkers by asking how many laps they've completed. (Typically, about half of the walkers come from outside our church, showing how the center has become a community venture.) "Older people especially need this," Loretta says. "We encourage them to come often, because the more they come, the better they feel—and the better they feel, the healthier they become."

Without question, the most noticeable result of our senior adult exercise programs has been the improvement in the overall health of our older members. I don't have an exact count, but I estimate that my trips to the hospital last winter were cut in half due to our folks being healthier and happier. This freed me up to do a number of other ministries. Now when I feel a need to visit with some of the older folks, I just go see them in the exercise center. Trust me, those visits are a lot more enjoyable than seeing someone in the hospital. These senior saints are certainly enjoying more of the abundant life Jesus talked about in John 10:10.

We've seen other exercise classes get going, too. In the winter of 2011, we started our first youth basketball league, with more than 100 children participating (if you haven't heard of Upward Sports, check out www.up ward.org). The first women's activity to get rolling was a women's dance/exercise class (I don't attend that one!). It got underway thanks to the initiative of member Kelly Napier. "It has given women who haven't exercised for a while a chance to get back at it," Kelly says. "There are mothers and daughters who have exercised together. It gets women together for camaraderie and to pray together. First we shared healthy recipes and had healthy snacks to give people an idea of what they could do. When it comes to eating, it's kind of up to the women because usually they're doing the grocery shopping and cooking. When the mother is healthy and feeling good, it affects the whole family."

Feed Them and They Will Come

Big Losers sparked other action as well. After the first class, the women who cook our Wednesday night dinners said maybe they should make our meals healthier, too. I want to give special recognition to Barbara Hicks, Jane Galloway, Alice Lee Ferguson and Barbara Robertson. Though well into their retirement years, these women were young enough to look at life in new ways. They took the initiative to search for more low-fat and more low-calorie dishes. Things only got better with Jamie Oliver's arrival. He and his staff showed them healthier cooking techniques like avoiding mayonnaise-based dressings by using Miracle Whip and mixing in yogurt. Today, instead of frying potatoes, they rub them lightly with oil and bake them. They make creative salads with low-cal dressing and such ingredients as walnuts, spinach, red lettuce and apples. (Try one and you won't return to the Golden Arches.)

After filming the final *Food Revolution* episode at our church, we used the following week's sneak preview to launch a program to provide healthy meals for the community. We offer made-from-scratch dinners on Wednesday nights for $10 per family. That's right—*per family*. That is cheaper than fast food and much healthier. It allows working mothers to avoid rushing through the drive-thru before coming to church. Many churches complain they cannot get families to mid-week services, but it is difficult for parents to cook and get kids to church on a school day. Offer a good, family-style meal and watch what kind of response that generates.

Think about the time when Jesus wanted to give a crowd the words of life, but they didn't have any food. So, He told His disciples, "You give them something to eat" (Luke 9:13). Any church can do this and see success, as long as they provide a tasty, healthy, low-cost meal. Such a program requires adequate volunteers and thoughtful planning, but your church can do this. After our first year, we had served thousands of dinners and seen participation in our children's mid-week activities more than double.

I try to continue this pattern at our monthly potluck dinners. Most people know about these free-for-alls where everyone brings a pan of food to share. If your church sponsors such meals, have your pastor encourage people to bring fruit, salads and healthy vegetable dishes. As I mentioned in Round 1, we still see fried chicken and mashed potatoes at our potlucks, but now healthier choices have joined the buffet line.

At your potlucks, place healthier foods at the head of the line. It is human nature for people to fill their plates with the first few things they see, which is why many restaurants place high-carb, cheaper foods at the front of buffet lines. Operators know people will take the junk instead of waiting to get to the more expensive, healthier choices. We simply employed this tactic in reverse. When we put salads and vegetables up front, people cleaned them out first. Plus, salads and veggies took up so much room on their plates that they had less space for the fattening items on down the line. There is something to be said for shrewdness (see Matt. 10:16).

Promotion, Promotion, Promotion

I don't know that Jamie Oliver would have ever heard about our church if it weren't for a young lady named Courtney Ballengee. When we began our programs, Courtney called national news outlets and told them her church was doing something about that infamous CDC report that garnered us the "unhealthiest city in the nation" moniker. As a result of her calls, dozens of news agencies called us to see what we were doing. It not only got a buzz going around town, but it also brought hope to a negative situation.

Every church needs to promote local opportunities for healthier living, even if other churches or community groups are sponsoring those events or programs. If the local hospital is offering free health screenings for the poor, don't you think that is something Jesus would promote? Besides, once your church gets the reputation of being health conscious and community-oriented, you will probably see some health-minded visitors on Sunday mornings. I guarantee that there are some gifted, passionate people in your city who are looking for a church where they can invest their energies.

So what does a cooperative spirit look like? Before the Huntington Health Revolution kicked off with a 90-day challenge at the start of 2011, we sent out a letter to churches in our community, encouraging them to join. We mentioned the initiative in weekly bulletins and included an online link for more information. The challenge included diet and exercise plans and spiritually based activities to promote better health. It concluded with a 5K run/walk through Huntington and a healthy food festival for participants. We even had a sign-up list at our church.

We also support a local food pantry. In the past, we collected food from our members, but the donations were often in the form of unhealthy processed foods that had a shelf life just short of the Jurassic era. Now we try to bring healthier options so the less fortunate in our communities aren't being inundated with foods that will only compound their challenging situations.

Churches can make other, subtle changes too. We started putting out fruit and other healthy foods during fellowship activities and serving fruit to children for Sunday morning snacks. After several months, we experimented by putting out a tray of cookies next to the fruit at a Christmastime activity. Showing how quickly children can be conditioned to make healthy choices, the fruit vanished long before the cookies did. We should have bought more fruit, but we didn't want to risk throwing it away. Oh we of little faith!

We took these steps in the spirit of offering alternatives, not imposing rules. I sometimes tease people who choose fattening foods, but there is only so much I can do. Enjoying a healthier life is a choice. As much as I want them to win the food fight, I can't browbeat people into changing what they eat or force them to exercise. However, by creating a culture of healthier choices around the church—taking every opportunity to set out fruit trays instead of donuts—we are communicating the message that God cares about their health.

While I don't preach every week on food and fitness, I do sprinkle frequent references to physical stewardship into messages or announcements. Why shouldn't I? Food merchants are in my church members' faces daily through advertising, billboards, coupons and direct mail. During one advertising campaign in 2010, I asked the congregation, "What's back?" Everyone replied in unison, "McRib!" I knew that, too, even though I rarely go to McDonald's. Why? Because of the incessant advertising on billboards and TV. If fast-food companies bombard people multiple times a day, what is wrong with my mentioning good health once a week?

It Starts at the Top

I have a friend who attends a megachurch in Southern California. She has a well-known pastor who has also been known to struggle with his weight. Though some members of the church had previously attempted to address the issue of healthy living, nothing ever really materialized. Then one day, the pastor was baptizing a number of people from his congregation. Due to his poor physical condition, he found himself out of breath. In addition, he realized that part of the reason he was working so hard during the baptisms was that many of those being baptized were also overweight. Thankfully for him and his entire congregation, the lights came on, and he became a major proponent of good nutrition. Before long, he was encouraging the entire church to join a 52-week "get healthy initiative."

I share this story not because it is an anomaly, but because it is typical of most church programs. If the pastor isn't passionate about an idea—if he isn't living out the ideal in his own life—then the congregation probably won't get it either. Consequently, when it comes to churches helping improve our nation's health, I believe it will be impossible without strong pastoral leadership. If there is any group that I want to read this book, it is our nation's spiritual leaders. To see church-wide change, pastors have to push this issue.

So, I would like to turn this discussion specifically towards pastors. After wading through this thicket myself, I can promise that if you address this topic, you will receive a rainbow of responses. If you speak the truth in love, and people get mad at you for *what* you say, that is *their* problem. However, if they get mad at you for *how* you say what you say, that is *your* problem. You must broach this subject with an ounce of truth and a pound of grace. People who struggle with obesity are aware of their problem without you heaping on guilt. Still, people in our congregation who succeeded in losing weight often told me they didn't want to let *me* down. As a church leader, you may not realize how much influence you have over the people in your congregation. God has placed you in a position to speak truth and grace into their lives. A good word may help keep someone's family together or literally save someone's soul.

You may be thinking, "I don't have time to lead a food revolution in my church. I have visits to make, sermons to prepare, meetings to attend, family responsibilities . . . I cannot do everything." You are right! God never intended you to do everything—or even to make the attempt. Ephesians 4:12-13 says that the task of church leaders is to equip and prepare people to do ministry. If the food chains that bind your church are to be broken, the action steps will come from the people in the pews.

Perhaps you noticed that many of our success stories emanated from someone in our congregation coming to me and suggesting a ministry or program to help address the problem. Some ideas focused on behavior modification, but most were about changing the *attitudes* of those who struggled with poor nutrition. This is where you come in. There is no better way to address attitudes and belief systems than through practical, biblical teaching on what it means to love God with all your strength. You *can* do this; just salt your words with a lot of grace.

Regardless of size, any church can take the same kinds of steps we have. You can encourage people to bring healthy alternatives to potluck dinners or form groups to provide accountability for weight loss. You may not have enough members to enroll 40 or 50 people in a Big Losers-type class, but you can find five.

Don't get me wrong. The point of joining this movement is not to turn your church into a health club. Our perspective rests on Scripture. We aren't doing this to lose weight, promote exercise, or even simply to broadcast a message of good health. We want to align our bodies with God's plan for our lives. As God's Spirit flows through your congregation, you will see how the power of a local church can transform the health habits of an entire community. If it has happened in the unhealthiest city in America, it can happen where you live as well. But don't stop at church. Carry the fight into your community. Read how Huntington does that in Round 8.

Questions for Discussion

1. Enough shoppers in Huntington asked about healthy foods that stores started devoting sections to them. What grassroots actions can you generate to change conditions where you live?
2. Does your church have a positive outlook on healthy food choices? What types of foods are being shared in your children's department? At your potlucks?
3. How could you tactfully encourage a culture of healthy eating in your congregation?
4. First Baptist of Kenova began its Big Losers groups with members who didn't have degrees or expertise in health and exercise. Who in your church or community group could lead a similar class? How could you help get a class like this going at your church?
5. What ideas did you glean from this round that may work in your church? Who can you enlist to help turn these ideas into a reality?
6. Do you think your pastor cares about people's physical health? Why or why not? If not, what can you do to help your pastor understand the scriptural mandate we have to honor God with our bodies (see 1 Cor. 6:20)?

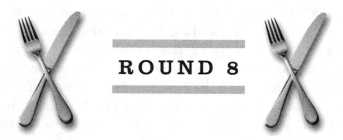

It's Taking a Village

When Yvonne Jones stood up to address the energized crowd that had crammed into the downtown Huntington restaurant, she had a specific message in mind. The executive director of Ebenezer Medical Outreach intended to inform residents that the ministry didn't have the resources to take over Jamie Oliver's kitchen once he concluded filming his mini-series. Instead, as the *Food Revolution* cameras rolled, she spontaneously declared, "The nation is looking at us. Let's let them see what a city can do when it decides to change and become the healthiest city in the nation instead of the fattest city in the nation."

Several months later, Ebenezer had the money. Cabell Huntington Hospital awarded a $50,000 grant to fund first-year operations at Jamie's cooking studio, which changed its name to Huntington's Kitchen. Still, Yvonne recognized that it would take more than healthy cooking classes to sustain the momentum created by the impending broadcasts. *Yvonne, if something's going to happen, somebody's going to have to do something,* she thought. Inspired, she got together with me, and we decided to invite people of influence in the community to an organizational meeting. Our vision was to form a taskforce that would promote the cause of healthy living long after the excitement of the mini-series had faded. Fifty people showed up for the first meeting; from that gathering emerged what we now call the Huntington Health Revolution.

Dividing into nine work groups—such as business, healthcare, publicity and civic/social organizations—the all-volunteer organization planned its first "90-Day Challenge." The program encourages residents to tackle changes in diet, exercise and spiritual life over a three-month period. For example, during week one, individuals are challenged to subtract a sugary drink (soda, Kool-Aid, sweet tea) daily and add a glass of water. For exercise, participants are exhorted to walk 30 minutes a day; and to bolster their spirits, they are encouraged to reserve five minutes for a daily quiet time.

At the conclusion of the first citywide challenge, the committee regrouped and organized a second challenge for the first three months of

2011. I have to be honest with you. The first challenge wasn't so successful, and we knew we had to do some things differently the second time around. In my opinion, our main failing was not getting the word out to the public about what we were doing.

The second event concluded with a walk/race downtown, followed by a health food festival and games at the city's main shopping and entertainment plaza. Even before the celebration that attracted nearly 200 runners to a 5K run and several hundred other participants, Yvonne knew these challenges were making an impact. "I used to walk in the park, and when I went there after the challenge started, I noticed more people walking than before," she says. "On one of my walks, I met a couple who said, 'Your 90-Day Challenge has us out here.' It gives people things they can do, like slowing down and taking it easy, cutting things like mayonnaise out of their diet, and changing some of their habits."

I don't know how long our taskforce will continue, but both Yvonne and I know the key to long-term change is addressing the food system in Huntington. One obstacle low-income people face is a lack of grocery stores stocking healthy items. The only food sources customarily within walking distance in low-income communities are convenience stores or fast-food outlets, leaving those without ready access to transportation with few alternatives to fattening diets.

Yvonne recognizes that sustaining momentum will be a challenge all its own. This is partially because of funding issues, and partially because no one entity has sole responsibility for promoting the Health Revolution. But that is why people like Yvonne Jones are critical to winning your community's food fight. It's not in her job description to find ways to get healthy food to low-income families; she just does it out of the goodness of her heart. "It seems like this is going to have to be an ongoing thing for a long, long time," Yvonne says. "We're talking about a generation of bad habits. It's going to be a long-term effort. This is not a short-term thing that lasts a month. We have to keep plugging away at it."

Making a Difference

There will always be challenges when you tackle the food fight in your city. People may ridicule your efforts or react with indifference and apathy. Vested interests in the food industry and others who depend on maintaining the status quo will raise sometimes-subtle opposition. The sheer busyness and hectic pace of life can easily sidetrack you. All of these issues are secondary to Rule #1: We have to change the dietary culture in the United States. This won't happen overnight, and it won't come easily. However, the concerted efforts of countless individuals will make a difference.

Don't think you must plan every step in advance. Things you never dreamed of will happen along the way. I never imagined a prayer for help with nutrition would lead to a call from Jamie Oliver's production company the next day. I also never imagined that someone like Jill Moore, who earned her law degree from Capital University in 2008, would put her legal career on hold to become the kitchen manager at Huntington's Kitchen. Jill and Yvonne were connected through their work at Ebenezer Medical Outreach, and Yvonne knew Jill had the skills to do the job. Yvonne asked. Jill responded.

This is one of the keys to getting things going in your community. Be passionate about Rule #1, convince those around you that things have to change, and then ask them to help be the change your community needs to see. Ten community leaders may tell you "no," but the one who says "yes!" may make more things happen than you could ever imagine.

By the way, don't be afraid to ask busy people to join your local task-force. My mom always told me, "If you want to get something done, ask a busy person to do it." Movers and shakers are always busy—because they have a drive to get things done. Yvonne Jones is a busy person. Jill Moore is a busy person. Our committee members are all busy people. But because they believe in what we are doing, they make the time to get things done.

Some of the most crucial people on our committee are folks who work on the funding of Huntington's Kitchen. Cabell Huntington Hospital has since donated another $100,000 to help fund the kitchen's second and third years of operations, which paid for the lease and utilities in 2011-2012. Beyond that, Jill says that whether the kitchen remains open depends on what grants and additional income Ebenezer can generate. Future concerns aside, opening and maintaining Huntington's Kitchen has required more than the hospital funding. Just converting the storefront space from a TV studio meant installing gas and electric lines and buying a commercial dishwasher and other equipment. That is where the village came into play. Much of the elbow grease needed for this changeover came from volunteers whose only reward was the satisfaction of helping. You'll need to raise up this kind of "people power" wherever you live.

"Funding is always going to be an issue," says Jill, who gave us two great years before departing last spring for a position in the legal profession. "If you're looking at a community set-up, you're not going to be able to say, 'I've already got a guaranteed source of funding' unless you charge $50 per cooking lesson. The key is to do it at a cost people in the community can afford. Communities can look at grants or find some supermarkets that want to support healthy eating initiatives."

Grants don't automatically mean government sources. In fact, in an era of soaring federal deficits and restricted state budgets, that may be the last place to look. However, there are foundations, nonprofit organizations, hospitals, churches and other groups that support healthy lifestyles. Groups such as the Catholic Diocese of Wheeling-Charleston, Sacred Heart, and St. Stephen Parish have made critical contributions to the cause. In 2010, Ebenezer secured a $25,000 grant from Share Our Strength, a Washington, DC-based non-profit whose goals include securing more healthy food for hungry children. That money supported a series of free "Cooking Matters" classes for low-income residents.

Huntington's Kitchen doesn't serve only low-income citizens. Its eight-week series of "Jamie Classes" are open to all at a cost of $10 per session. Since the kitchen can only accommodate 12 students at a time, its impact is quietly rippling through the region. During its first seven months, 375 people came through the doors. Of those, 185 graduated and another 50 participated in at least three classes. The remainder includes travelers who have dropped in for individual sessions. We encourage them to go back home and try to begin a similar movement in their cities.

"Part of what Jamie's kitchen is all about is you passing it on and teaching other people," says Jill, who emphasizes that any community can start healthy cooking classes with a minimum of equipment and expertise. Jill has "passed on" her responsibilities to Andi Leffingwell, who is doing a great job of inviting community groups into the kitchen. "I'm in touch with several people who are still doing healthy cooking and have taught their mother or sister, so I feel we've made an impact on people's eating habits," says Jill. "Lots of people have said, 'You made a difference. I look at nutrition labels now, and if I can't pronounce something, I don't buy it.' Calories and fat are not our focus. As Jamie says, it's about eating more natural food. If you improve the quality of the food you eat, you will be healthier."

Looking for a Green Thumb

Community gardens have found new life here and offer similar promise to your community. The amazing story of how the gardens returned to life in Huntington involves coordinator Jennifer Williams and her leading helper, Eve Marcum-Atkinson, and is another illustration of my earlier comment that as you step into the arena of healthy living, things you never dreamed possible will take place.

A month after the release of the CDC report, Jennifer was in the midst of graduate studies at Marshall University. Battling some personal problems, she often went to the downtown riverfront park to pray. One day the phrase "community gardens" floated through her mind. That caused her to scoff, "No way, that's ridiculous. I don't have time, and I don't know how to grow anything." Still, she couldn't shake the idea. That led to a conversation with sociology professor Vaughn Grisham, director of a community development institute at the University of Mississippi, who visited Huntington that year to consult with local officials on ways of capitalizing on the area's intrinsic assets. While in town, Grisham also brought increased visibility to the work of Create Huntington, a volunteer-driven organization that has spurred numerous positive developments and makes small grants to help visionaries develop their ideas to better the city.

Jennifer's next step was meeting with participants in Create Huntington. That led to sending an email to Eve, who had blogged about community gardens on the group's website. Jennifer and Eve met in mid-February 2009. Two months later, the pair had acquired lots on three different sites, including land next to a neighborhood center that houses a branch office of the police department. On Earth Day, the governor of West Virginia attended the ribbon cutting for the revitalized program. Three days before the ceremony, while surveying the muddy lot where it would be held, Jennifer had looked up and said, "God, we need some sod." The next day, the manager of a Lowe's in eastern Kentucky called to say, "We have 19 rolls of sod. Could you use that?"

Other assistance materialized as well. Besides the free sod, the program obtained a cargo van, use of a greenhouse, a tiller, an office, more lots, hundreds of volunteers and numerous supplies. This activity generated additional gardens, with volunteers offering their expertise. The program began lending garden implements to churches and schools. To complete the picture, the year after the ribbon-cutting ceremony, Jennifer was hired as an extension associate by West Virginia State University. Her new position included teaching nutrition classes and improving residents' knowledge of healthy eating. That put her in the perfect place to continue coordinating the gardens. With the help of another extension agent, Melissa Stewart, and her Junior Master Gardener program, the Huntington Community Gardens gained viability after only two years. Things were going so well that Jennifer applied for another grant that would enable her to hire four more people to help run this growing ministry. She knew it was a long shot, but as I said earlier, you have to ask. Thank God, Jennifer got the grant, and now our community garden project will continue for years to come.

Community gardens are an idea whose time has come. They are necessary because the more we have industrialized our food system, the less nutritious our produce has become. We all know that produce from a local farm tastes better than vegetables that have been genetically altered, grown in nutrient-deficient soils, cultivated with artificial fertilizers, doused with pesticides, over-saturated with water to increase their weight at market, and plucked off the vine weeks before they are ripe. But that's not the worst of it. Studies are demonstrating that these non-organic farms are turning out vitamin-deficient produce.[1] The result is that when you buy "fresh" tomatoes at the store, they may not be providing the nutrients tomatoes are supposed to provide. Granted, even non-organic fruits and vegetables are better than processed junk and fast food, but if you're striving for the best, you need to budget for organic produce—or, even better, grow your own. (If neither of these is an option, we'll talk about vitamin supplements later in this round.)

The American Community Gardening Association (www.community garden.org) has numerous resources and tips on starting a garden in your city. Our church signed up for one last year with the hope of teaching our kids more about food and helping them acquire a taste for fresh vegetables.

When you get kids in a garden for the first time, they'll tell you some funny things. "Our second summer, while we were at one of the gardens in public housing, I heard one boy say, 'Those cucumbers look like pickles,'" Jennifer says. "Like I did as a child, many of the kids we work with thought vegetables just came from the grocery store. The kids are so much more likely to try new foods if they grow it themselves. Volunteers who come have access to the food, and any overage is used in nutrition classes. It's exciting to show people how they can pick fresh tomatoes and cook tomato soup straight out of the garden."

During 2011, one of my favorite adventures was a cooperative effort involving our church, some college students, and the community garden movement. During a sermon, I threw out the idea for a community garden, and I quickly found dozens of volunteers. A handful of people offered their land. We wound up with two projects, one in the country and the other in the inner city.

To those who consider God a mythical figure or an abstract concept, consider what transpired that spring. Member Marcia Wilson came from a family that values nutrition. She and her mother often made three-hour trips to Columbus, Ohio, just to visit Whole Foods. When I prayed one Sunday, "Lord, give us some land so we can grow healthy food," Marcia had an epiphany. "I had prayed that morning and said, 'God, what can I do to help this area get healthier?'" she told me afterward. "So when you asked for help, I nearly jumped out of my seat!"

Marcia had two acres of land and plenty of farming equipment to get us started. Within weeks we had volunteers planting seeds, and they were excited about harvesting healthy crops. By the time August arrived, we had more food than we could eat. I cannot tell you the joy we received as the children from our church raced into the produce-filled garden like it was a giant Easter egg hunt. They were eating raw corn off the stalk and loving it. "This is the best food I've ever tasted!" exclaimed one youngster.

We heard similar stories from other families. The same children who hated vegetables one year earlier had suddenly turned into natural food enthusiasts. They participated in the planting and growing process, knew where the food came from, and developed an appreciation for how it arrived on their plates. As a result, they found dinnertime much more interesting than when it meant opening a can of stale green beans and choking down processed meat.

Our other garden near a low-income housing project proved equally successful. Some of our college students, led by Kyle Baughman, took the time to plant and cultivate that garden. As they were heading home for the summer, Kyle let some of the community residents know that once the vegetables were ripe, they were welcome to come into the garden and take whatever they liked. "I had no idea if anyone would take us up on the offer, but it was worth a try," Kyle said. "Nobody signed up, and we never put up a sign or anything, but people seemed receptive to the idea."

I never learned exactly how many families took advantage of Kyle's offer, but every time I went to check, most of the ripened food had vanished—which is what we wanted. The neighbors were happy to get fresh produce; we just had to make it accessible to them. Our goal is to multiply the number of churches and community groups who will take plots of unused land like this in the city, develop a garden, and allow residents to pick all the vegetables they can use. We generated a buzz, and we want to keep it going!

By the way, we had so much food left over from Marcia's land that we couldn't give it all away to people from our church. So I did a sociological experiment. I had routinely heard that disadvantaged people didn't like healthy food—that they would rather eat junk out of a can than cook fresh vegetables. So I took four bushels of fresh green beans to our community food pantry and set them by the door. I planned to record what percentage of needy families took the fresh beans instead of cans lining the shelves (both of which were free). I quickly realized that I wouldn't have to count too closely. Every single person who came in not only chose the fresh food but also all smiled excitedly and expressed gratitude. One mother said, "I'd much rather have this stuff than that canned junk. Why won't the government give us options like this?"

At first, that was exactly my perception. However, the more I pondered her statement, the more I understood that winning this food fight won't originate with Washington, DC. While it sure would help if the federal government considered more subsidies for fresh fruits and vegetables (more on that in Round 10), the power of community gardens is within our grasp. This is literally a grass-roots campaign that can happen in your subdivision *this* spring. Don't wait for Uncle Sam to come in and save the day. Join with like-minded individuals and provide fresh produce for your community. Sure, you may make a few mistakes, but so did we. Now that we have learned from them, we cannot wait to do it again. If a bunch of unorganized yahoos and college students can make this work, you can too!

Running for Your Life

Eating quality food is only half the battle. We need community organizations that focus on exercise as well. Pat Riley discovered that when he attended Marshall University. A graduate of Cabell Midland High School, where he now teaches business education, Pat had been a runner as a teen. Like many students, he got overwhelmed by the demands of college courses and stopped working out. That, coupled with a poor diet, resulted in a 75-pound weight gain. However, during his senior year, a friend taught him good nutrition, and he resumed regular workouts. That combination has helped Pat drop more than 65 pounds since 2005.

Running has become like a second job for Pat (or a third, if you count his position as track coach). He is such an avid runner that in 2007 he set up TriStateRacer.com, which spotlights local races as well as regional and national events. Given his experience and interest in running, Pat found the 2008 Centers for Disease Control report disturbing. He thought, *How have things gotten so bad in my hometown?* He sensed dismay brewing among citizens, and he acknowledges that at first he felt the same way.

"I think Huntington went through all seven," Pat says of the classic stages of grief, which start with denial and continue through such emotions as anger and guilt before concluding with acceptance. "We all needed a little bit of time to think about it and process the report. I think finally we accepted it and said, 'Okay, but we should do something about it.' That December, I lay in bed one night and couldn't sleep. Finally, I thought, *Let's do the biggest road race West Virginia has ever seen.* The 'fattest city in America' label was a big motivation to do it."

Setting out to find an interested partner, Pat persuaded United Way of the River Cities to help organize the West Virginia 5K Championship. Previously, the state's largest race had been the "Bun Run" that coincides with the annual West Virginia Hot Dog Festival in late July. In 2008, the Bun Run had 350 contestants. The first West Virginia 5K in June 2009 attracted 519, and participation increased to 541 the next year. Equally impressive is the number of races now held throughout the region. Tri StateRacer.com tracks events across West Virginia and about 75 miles into eastern Kentucky and southern Ohio. Though numbers fluctuate, there are around 125 races annually. Except during the winter (when outdoor events are fewer and farther between), there's at least one race nearly every weekend.

There is undoubtedly a running fraternity in your city, and within that community you will likely find untapped resources—people who are quietly making a difference. Enlist their support in your efforts—for instance, by calling on them to speak to school groups, civic organizations or church-based seminars.

In late 2010, I heard about a man who was working to create a community-wide ministry that hopes to one day operate a fitness camp in this area. Mickey Bane started Fit4Life Ministries after a long-time struggle with his health. Due to his battle with obesity, he had major lung problems, which prevented the family from becoming missionaries to England. His daughter grew so upset that she temporarily stopped speaking to him. Depressed and thinking he had failed God, Mickey escaped into food. Already heavy from constant overeating during travels to raise financial support for the mission field, by the summer of 2006 he peaked at 304 pounds.

Things turned around when his daughter told him he was going to take her on a mission trip the following summer. If he didn't lose 100 pounds, she warned, he had to pay all the expenses. So, Mickey joined the YMCA, where at first all he could do was tread water. Over the next year, he worked his way up to running, weight lifting and cardiovascular training. In the process of researching nutrition, Mickey discovered that he needed to adjust his food intake as well. "The more I read, the more I realized it was about eating balanced meals," he says. "It wasn't just about counting calories, but looking at food as fuel for daily life. I didn't follow a diet. I just put together the healthiest food program I could. I consumed a lot of raw vegetables, lean protein and fruit."

Before I share the rest of Mickey's story, I'd like to point out that his dietary advice is right on the mark. Getting healthy is not so much about a dietary plan, but a plan for a healthier diet. As Michael Pollan states in the bestselling *In Defense of Food,* the key to health is as simple as seven words: "Eat food. Not too much. Mostly plants."[2] That is a positive way of saying, "Don't eat processed junk. Stay away from manufactured sugars and fats. Eat things that God had growing on earth before we humans got involved. Eat until you are satisfied, but not until you feel 'full.'" (If you eat the right amount, the full feeling will come about 20 minutes after you stop eating.)

Mickey's life parallels the other personal accounts in this book: When he got his eating under control, it affected other areas of his life. Doctors had told him he would need lung medications forever, but after losing 110 pounds he no longer needed them. Academically, he buckled down and got his credentials at the American College of Sports Medicine so he could run his own fitness program. Although Fit4Life has been a part-time endeavor, in 2011 Mickey completed paperwork to make it a federally registered non-profit. Though he never made it to England, today Mickey makes it his mission in life to teach both physical and spiritual health to anyone who will listen. From my vantage point, that's a mission field too.

Remember the Media

An important ally in the fight against fat is local news media. In today's often-fractious political environment, too many draw "us vs. them" lines when it comes to media, forgetting that newspapers, radio and TV stations, and magazines offer a valuable public service. Health is a prime topic of ongoing news coverage in our area. The NBC affiliate here not only airs more than a dozen news stories a week, but it also arranged, in 2009, to produce a local version of the network's hit show, *Biggest Loser*. The Fox network station (owned by the same company that manages the ABC outlet) hired a reporter specifically to cover stories prompted by the *Food Revolution*. Huntington's daily newspaper, *The Herald-Dispatch*, has produced thousands of stories on health over the past decade, both in news and editorial columns. In 2009, the newspaper's coverage won an award for public service from the West Virginia Press Association.

Herald-Dispatch editor Ed Dawson has been an incredible ally in our local fight against obesity. He has observed that obesity spills over into numerous issues of health, nutrition, environment and public policy, meaning that the newspaper has no shortage of things to write about. In addition, *The Herald-Dispatch* has circulated information about lifestyle adjustments individuals and groups can make, as well as exercise initiatives, such as the Paul Ambrose Trail for Health. This still-developing series of hiking and bicycle paths is named for a former Marshall student and promising young physician. Dr. Ambrose had just edited a surgeon general's report about reducing obesity when the plane he was on crashed into the Pentagon during the 9-11 terrorist attacks.

"I think the community is beginning to see, after they've gotten a lot more information about this, that in addition to being an individual decision there are a lot of societal decisions that have to be made," Dawson says. "Food in the schools is one of those. There are many. Making changes on a policy level will help everyone with the problem. On the other side, there are a lot of good things going on, and people are realizing they have to look at things in a new way. There's a lot of good that has come from this discussion. It's just not going to be something that is going to change overnight."

The Economic Incentive

Another aspect of our village coming together may surprise you. After doing the New York publicity tour and being on Jamie's show, I received over

200 emails, phone calls and letters from various companies wanting me to endorse their products. We had so many calls to the church, my secretary asked for extra help in the front office! I had offers for everything from healthy coffees and frozen produce to organic chocolate and natural sugar. I even had a chiropractor offer me a one-year lease on a BMW if I'd be in one of his commercials. I thought, *Some of those TV evangelists might get away with this, but that wouldn't fly in West Virginia!*

I won't mislead you. I talked to a number of companies; but even though some of them had interesting products and made generous offers for my family, I couldn't see how being involved with any of them would benefit our church. I've seen too many pastors ruin their credibility by chasing after a dollar, so I decided to walk away from everything.

But that's when a friend introduced me to a company in California whose CEO has family ties to our area. This CEO, Ryan Blair, had seen us on ABC. Because of his personal connection to Huntington, he wanted to help us however he could. His multi-million dollar company, ViSalus Sciences, distributes nutrient- and protein-rich meal replacement shakes, vitamins, and a herb-based energy drink. "I still feel connected to Huntington," he told me when we first spoke. "If we can do something to help kids get the nutrition they need, you let me know." I was waiting for the sales pitch or the catch, but there wasn't one. He didn't ask me to endorse the company or be in any commercials. He just wanted to help because he had once been a kid on a school lunch program, and he could remember not being able to get decent nutrition when he was a child. He was offering us hundreds of their shakes that are loaded with vitamins and contain almost no sugars or simple carbohydrates.

Granted, I'm not a nutritionist, and to a certain extent it sounded too good to be true. However, I was intrigued enough to check out ViSalus Sciences' website to see what they were about. I was pleased to see that helping children was not something new for Ryan Blair. While on a trip to Kingston, Jamaica, he had witnessed malnourished youngsters who were suffering because of the nation's drug-related crime and other social problems. "I thought, *There's got to be a way economically that we can create a sustained impact and not just be charitable and distribute our gains,*" Ryan says. "We are a community, and we formed a mission to give meal replacements to kids who can't afford to have the right nutrients in their diets. In some cases, they can't even afford to put on weight. In each community where we launch ViSalus, we look to set up ties to charities, churches and organizations to distribute meals so our distributors can make an impact alongside the company."

Although skeptics would point to Blair's status as a rich entrepreneur and scoff, "It's all about money," for him it goes deeper. After his father abandoned them when Ryan was 13 years old, he and his mother moved into a low-income housing development north of Los Angeles. Although his mother worked seven days a week, her modest salary meant they had to subsist on macaroni and cheese and other fatty government commodities. At his peak, Ryan (who weighs around 190 today) ballooned to 260 pounds. Besides being sensitive to those who can't afford to eat better, he has a heart for at-risk youngsters who are facing the kind of circumstances he did as a teen. He knows what it is like to be labeled as "dysfunctional" or "suffering from ADD" (attention deficit disorder) just because a child is suffering from a lack of proper nutrition.

"Having been poor and eaten poor, now I love quality food," Ryan says. "I love eating correctly. I believe in a balanced approach and enjoying food. I enjoy food, but I also believe in exercise and vitamin supplements. If you have a combination of all those, you can have a life you enjoy better."

As I learned more about Ryan's ideas for a community partnership, it made sense for us to connect to his initiative. Ryan flew to West Virginia to help launch our area's first 90-day challenge at First Baptist of Kenova. He also presented our church with a check for $12,000—enough to purchase 30,000 child-size shakes (the check was symbolic; the company later shipped us the shake packets). Since that time, ViSalus distributors have donated over $30,000 worth of product for our local and international ministries. We continue to work with local food pantries to provide low-income families with healthier foods, but we also understand that many of the commodities they receive from the government do not give them the nutrients they need. In situations like these, diets must be supplemented with vitamins and fiber, or the children from these families will not develop the way God intended.

I share the ViSalus story for three reasons. First, the company's executives have taught me that if you tie financial or other material benefits to physical health, people respond. Each year, ViSalus rewards a cruise to the distributors who have had the biggest health turnarounds. In addition, employees have a built-in economic incentive: If they can't demonstrate that their product has helped them slim down, they can't expect others to try it. The lack of perceived economic incentive is a major contributor to the problem we have with the types of foods we eat—people are convinced that eating junk saves them money. They believe that something off the dollar menu will fill them up, so they take the cheapest option. Fruits and vegetables cost more than a bag of chips, so guess what they give their kids for a snack? That's right: diabetes in a bag.

To change our communities, we have to communicate to the masses that eating poorly does NOT save you much money, and it will also cost you thousands of dollars in the future. Poor nutrition in adults leads to poor performance at work. If you don't produce at work, you likely won't get a bonus, a raise or a promotion. When kids don't eat well at school, it affects their ability to learn—which, over time, will affect their ability to get a good job and earn a decent wage. Simply stated, they will not be all they can be if they don't eat like they're supposed to eat.

In addition, eating poorly costs money in medical bills, prescriptions, visits to the doctor . . . do you see my point? It's "pay me now or pay me later." We either put our financial support behind our bodies now (through good nutrition), or we'll pay 10 times that amount later due to increased medical costs. The choice is ours.

The second reason I share this story is that I believe there are hundreds of Ryan Blairs out there. If you tell the businesses in your community that you are doing something to improve the health of the children in their own backyard, many of them will respond. Go in to them with a plan, present the need, and ask for help. The worst they can do is tell you no—and my personal experience has been that most people *want* to help; they just don't know *how* to help.

Finally, as I mentioned earlier, I believe it is important to supplement your diet with vitamins, especially if you are unable to purchase large amounts of organic produce. The reality of our nation's current food system is that even when we eat our meats, grains, fruits and vegetables, because of the way the food is produced, those items do not supply all the vitamins and minerals our bodies need for proper development. My wife is somewhat of a purist when it comes to whole foods and nutrition, but no matter how we altered our youngest son's diet, he still struggled mightily with ADHD. Without question, removing sugary drinks and cutting out junk food made him better, but Lucas still struggled. We refused to put him on mind-altering medications, but apparently diet alone wasn't going to take care of the problem.

One day I was sharing our situation with David Stuart, one of ViSalus's national directors and a Huntington resident, and he suggested I give my son some of their Omega-3 supplements. We didn't see an overnight change, but now that Lucas has been on the Omegas for a while, my wife swears by them. He is a different child. I wonder how many children in your community would have their lives changed if they just had the nutrition they need. This is why our school lunch programs are so important, and why we, as community leaders, have to take our cause to the next level. We start with the schoolhouse in Round 9.

Questions for Discussion

1. When your church or community group starts a project, how do you go about the planning? Do you allow for the kind of unexpected help that Yvonne Jones, Jill Moore and Jennifer Williams experienced? Why or why not?

2. Has your church or organization ever investigated grants to fund a worthwhile community project? Who are some community leaders that might be willing to assist you in writing up a proposal for a grant?

3. Do any community gardens exist in your area? How could you join this initiative or start one yourself?

4. How can you enlist local media to assist in spreading the word about good nutrition?

5. Who are the Ryan Blairs of your community? How can you go to them and enlist their support?

6. How can we best communicate to our communities that taking care of our bodies will lead to economic benefits in the future?

7. What assistance does your community provide to ensure that local children are getting proper nutrition? If there aren't any such programs, what can you do to get something started?

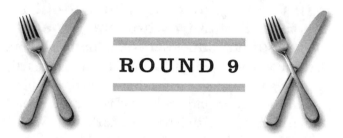

ROUND 9

Back to School

April Hamilton's initiation into the bureaucracy standing in the way of healthier school lunches occurred in the fall of 2007 when she joined the wellness committee of her child's middle school. April quickly discovered that some school groups' favorite fundraising activities involved selling pizza and donuts—a habit that clashed with her sensibilities. Having taught nutrition and cooking classes professionally since 2003, she regularly instructs students in Charleston, West Virginia, through "April's Kitchen." April has also taught kids' cooking classes at Huntington's Kitchen.

As parents and staff members discussed raising funds to support extracurricular activities, April asked if they could sell fruit smoothies. Pro football star and West Virginia native Randy Moss had started a shop that would deliver them in coolers for fund-raisers. When the principal said that might conflict with their contract with a soft drink manufacturer, "I'm sure smoke poured from my ears," April recalls. That incident sparked meetings with the cooks at an elementary school, the county's coordinator of child nutrition, and state education officials.

This marriage of business interests and our public schools is nothing new. I know from working with our local schools that most are so strapped for funding that they regularly accept assistance from local beer distributors. Obviously we aren't going to promote alcohol in our schools (then again, maybe that day will come), but soda companies are shameless when it comes to promoting their products to children. I'll never forget the time I solicited a local soda distributor to help us with a high school after-prom activity. They generously offered $500, on the condition that we display banners promoting their sugar-filled product in feeder schools. Not knowing any better at the time, we took the money.

Don't think this is unique to West Virginia. Have you ever wondered why most of the business "partnerships" we see in our schools are somehow related to sugar, fat and salt? Writes Dr. Marion Nestle, a professor in the department of nutrition, food studies and public health at New York

University, "Given their purchasing power, numbers, potential as future customers, and captive status, it is no wonder that food companies view schoolchildren as an unparalleled marketing opportunity."[1] On her website (www.foodpolitics.com), Dr. Nestle offers hundreds of examples of the food industry exerting influence over government agencies to gain an advantage in the nation's food fight.

What does this look like on the local level? For April Hamilton, it meant a series of dead-end meetings that extended over a three-year period. Her situation illustrates a reality inherent in school food issues: Parents and other activists must be in it for the long haul, because otherwise the bureaucracy will wear them down. April admits that she sometimes gets frustrated with the snail's pace of change and the apathy she encounters. Still, she believes that reforming menus is worth the effort.

"I realized something had to be done," April says. "This has nothing to do with my children, since they all pack some kind of lunch. I'm trying to help others who don't have healthy lunches to eat at school. Last year I went to school and saw sugar-frosted flakes and non-dairy whipped topping in the kitchen. What dietary food group is whipped topping in? It's full of hydrogenated oils."

April was particularly frustrated because that experience took place after a visit to Kanawha County (in which Charleston is located) by Connecticut-based Sustainable Food Systems (SFS) in October 2010. This is the same consulting firm that helped Cabell County's schools make the transition to healthier menus during and after Jamie Oliver's visit. After talking with SFS President John Turenne, April suggested that Kanawha County ask him to evaluate its procedures. The school board agreed to the idea, and April formed an ad hoc group she dubbed "Launching a New Lunch." Illustrating what a couple of passionate citizens can accomplish, in a few weeks she and fellow advocate Carol Spann raised $13,000 to cover the expenses of the consultation.

After SFS presented its recommendations (and most everyone liked their ideas), April encountered delays trying to get approval for a follow-up pilot program. Excuses given for the slowdown were new personnel, a once-every-five-years state audit, weather-related school closings, and other issues. As a result, instead of the pilot study being completed during the 2010-2011 school year, it got pushed back to 2011-2012 at the earliest.

Such delays, coupled with resistance to change, can frustrate parents and other well-intentioned community members who want their tax dollars put to better use. Still, everyone pushing for healthy food must remember the value of small, incremental changes. The three schools in April's vicinity now have salad bars, and the local elementary school has a small garden where she grows, picks and cleans baby organic lettuce. April's produce winds up on children's plates, where it helps create an impression that will outlast one day's meal.

Avoiding Conflict

Since I'm one of the people who advised April to make a little more noise if she hoped to see change, I can't fault her for her sometimes-outspoken efforts to keep this issue in front of the school board. Even so, as parents and others push for action, it is important to avoid adopting an "us vs. them" mentality or engaging in shouting and name calling, which drive officials into a defensive corner. John Turenne is familiar with how such an approach is likely to fail. Prior to forming his consulting firm in 2005, he spent 25 years as a chef and food service director, most recently at Yale University.

John came to Huntington in the fall of 2009 to help Jamie Oliver design lunch menus and advise school personnel about using more vegetables, salads and other fresh ingredients. He says reactions his team received in West Virginia were similar to those they've experienced in other states. In general, when they arrive at kitchens before sun-up on a Monday morning, if the local cooks' eyes could speak, they would say, "What's going on? Who are you, where are you from, and why are you here? What are you going to do to me? Why do I need to change?" However, by Friday afternoon, cooks are sharing photos of their grandchildren, exchanging email addresses and hugs, and saying things like, "Thank you. This is what needs to happen. You made me realize it can happen here."

"That respectful, empathetic, knowledgeable approach is how we can get involved," John says. "But when you have a group of advocates like parents at the gates, pounding on things and saying, 'You've got to stop serving this and serve something else!' it just builds walls. The reason it works in our model is because we go into things in a holistic manner. It's not only about changing the food. We have to look at five different factors; food is only one."

John compares these five factors to the spokes needed to enable a bicycle to run smoothly. Naturally, the first is food, which includes the ingredients—how the food is grown or raised and where it comes from—as well as recipes, menus and related issues. The remaining factors are:

- *Facilities.* This includes equipment, storage space, and other items used to prepare and serve the food.

- *Community.* This is all personnel involved, whether cooks, managers, administrators, students, parents or external experts, such as area chefs who can lend their time, energy and expertise.

- *Communication.* This is how change agents get their message across. Ideally these efforts will help personnel understand not only why change is desirable, but also the philosophy behind it.

- *Fiscal responsibility.* Change can't come, particularly in this financially distressed age, unless it is fiscally responsible and adheres to U.S. Department of Agriculture (USDA) guidelines. Monitoring costs and meeting federal guidelines are musts.

The good news on this final point is that the USDA is reforming some of its practices. After much ado and last-minute political wrangling, Congress finally got on board to pass the Healthy, Hunger-Free Kids Act of 2010. (From someone who communicated closely with a number of behind-the-scenes proponents of this bill, I can tell you that it did not go through without a fight. The final vote doesn't show it, but special interests nearly killed the bill just days before the end of the 111th Congress.) Thankfully, these guidelines will eventually impose limits on calories in student lunches and require schools to offer more fruits and vegetables, not just corn and potatoes. There are also provisions to assist local schools in starting community gardens so children can eat food they grow themselves.

"Where those guidelines will help is getting the food companies and these major brands on board, making changes to the ingredients they're putting in food," John says. "Is it enough? That's where I say 'no.' We still need to look at learning to cook food again—not just heating up food-like products. I'm talking about the entire United States school food program. What does it take to provide a lot of food to a lot of people with a minimal amount of hands to prepare it? Highly processed, heat-and-serve food. I challenge you to go into some of these places and see what they're serving, especially at breakfast. At times I shake my head. What is approved by the USDA as a meal sometimes blows my mind."

It shouldn't surprise him. John knows full well the battle that goes on in Washington. In the next round, I will share with you some of the intricacies of our nation's food politics. When we talk about school lunches, the two cannot be separated. Changing the way our schools deal with food depends on changing the way our government deals with food.

I am convinced that there are good people in the USDA and the Federal Drug Administration (FDA). Occasionally, a well-meaning agent attempts to make instructions about unhealthy foods more understandable for the average citizen. However, then the industrial food lobby flexes its muscle and halts language that addresses a specific food.[2] Instead of clearly stating that one of the keys to reducing obesity is *eating less* meat, dairy and eggs, our regulatory agencies—with their arms twisted behind their backs—agree to such abstract, ambiguous statements as: "We should practice moderation when it comes to fats, cholesterols, sugars, and salts."[3] Think about it—even when it comes to alcohol usage, when is the last time you heard the government encourage us to "eat less" or "drink less" of anything?

There are two major problems to this approach. One stems from the general public's lack of education about food and where it comes from. Because of this, most people have no idea about the fat loaded in our meats, the overabundance of salt in our chips, and the sugar stuffing our sodas and flavored school milks. We know these products have these ingredients, but according to our government, as long as we eat them "in moderation" we'll be fine. That leads to my second point. After a generation of manipulative advertising, many Americans have no idea what "moderation" means.[4] They equate moderation with only two trips through the buffet line instead of three or four.

Don't think for a second that the food industry isn't aware of all of this. In 1999, the USDA attempted to improve the national guidelines for food. In September 1999, the proposed language said to "go easy" on specific foods that make us fat and unhealthy. The food lobby got wind of the changes—and the next draft said we should "choose to limit" our intake of certain foods. By the time the guidelines emerged in May 2000, the "choose moderation" line had been reinserted. Can you see how the language manipulates the message? Instead of being encouraged to drink less soda, our government tells us to consume it "in moderation." Think about that for a minute. Why should our government encourage us to drink soda at all? Is it one of the four basic food groups? Is it *that* nutritious for our children? What we need to see from our friends in Washington are statements like, "If you struggle with obesity, we encourage you to *eliminate* sugary drinks from your diet." Maybe someday someone in our nation's capital will summon the political courage to make such a statement, but I'm not holding my breath.

Foxes in the Henhouse

In my opinion, at the root of the problem are the very purpose statements of the USDA and FDA. In many respects, their areas of oversight overlap. Priorities for the Secretary of Agriculture (the head of the USDA) include areas such as food production, international food trade, agribusiness, nutritional awareness and food safety.[5] The Food and Drug Administration is charged with protecting the public health.[6] I think you can see the potential for a conflict of interest. What happens when proper education about food steers people away from certain industries? For instance, what if we discover that high-fructose corn syrup and other corn derivatives have a relationship with heart disease? Or what if we realize that the flood of antibiotics we are giving our livestock reduces the effectiveness of other antibiotics in humans? While public safety would demand a drastic response—such as a halt in production of these items—what if this would mean the loss of thousands of jobs, and farmers and pharmaceutical companies losing billions of dollars?

The problem is only compounded when the former president of the National Cattlemen's Association is made chief of the USDA's Food Marketing and Inspection Division. (This happened in the 1990s![7]) Would it seem appropriate to you if a former executive in the pharmaceutical industry were placed in charge of the division of the FDA entrusted with overseeing the safety of prescription drugs?

I can see both sides of this issue. On the one hand, it's beneficial for someone from within the industry to oversee regulations because those on the inside know the "tricks of the trade." A former CEO of a large soybean company will likely know his or her industry better than someone from the outside. On the other hand, this very experience may inhibit the regulators. After all, if they are keeping these industries in check, they are likely to alienate many of the executives who were once their best friends. Tougher regulation usually means higher costs of production, and companies don't like that.

On a related note, while I do want to be careful not to be overly suspicious of government officials, it should concern all of us that the same group overseeing a food industry that is killing us is also overseeing the pharmaceutical companies that are getting rich from medicating us. What will happen to companies producing cholesterol medications if we all lose enough weight to stop taking those prescriptions? What will happen to the dairy industry if we take flavored, sugar-filled milk out of our school lunch programs? For that matter, why does the USDA order more milk when dairy prices go down? Does the amount of milk our children need rise and fall based on milk production?

While the Healthy, Hunger-Free Kids Act was a start, we still have a long way to go. Besides, just because laws and policies are passed, there is no guarantee they will be implemented. As a study at the University of Chicago demonstrated, citizens must remain vigilant when it comes to school lunches. In 1995, after research showed that many school lunches failed to meet nutrition requirements, Congress passed an initiative to provide healthy meals. The policy required that food served in school cafeterias meet one-third of a child's daily recommended allowance of calories, protein, calcium, iron, and vitamins A and C, and contain a maximum of 30 percent of calories from fat. This was a good start! Yet a decade later, only 4 percent of public schools met all the guidelines outlined in the congressional bill. So, although it's encouraging that Congress again acted in 2010 to improve the situation, we cannot act as if the problems will be resolved overnight (or without our continued involvement).

Realistically it will take awhile for guidelines issued in January 2011 to make it to your local school system, but keep abreast of the progress of these changes and make sure your school takes advantage of the Healthy, Hunger-Free Kids Act of 2010.

Criticizing School Lunches

School lunches attract a fair amount of criticism, particularly after a study released in 2010. Published in the *American Heart Journal*, the five-year-long review of approximately 1,000 sixth-graders at several schools in southeastern Michigan found that children who regularly ate school lunches were 29 percent more likely to be obese than those who brought lunch from home. "Most school lunches rely heavily on high-energy, low-nutrient-value food, because it's cheaper," said Dr. Kim Eagle, director of the University of Michigan Cardiovascular Center. Dr. Eagle pointed out that some schools offer specials like "Tater Tot Day" to keep costs down.[8]

Obesity among children ages 6 to 11 has increased at an alarming rate over the past three decades, tripling from 6.5 percent in 1980 to 19.6 percent in 2008. However, to take the news about the Michigan study as evidence that school lunches are solely to blame is to oversimplify a serious societal problem. The Michigan study notes that obese children also spend two hours a day watching TV or playing video games. Dr. Eagle states that genetic screening may be a consideration for extremely overweight children, but for the rest, increasing physical activity and reducing recreational screen time are vital.

We, as parents, clearly have an important role to play—not only in taking responsibility for our children getting sufficient exercise, but also in dealing with the uncomfortable truth of our own eating habits. School lunch programs can be a convenient scapegoat, but they are by no means the whole problem. New York author Jane Black—whose book about Huntington's eating habits is due out in 2013—recognizes this issue. In an article about the Michigan study, she notes that it is easy to forget that improved school nutrition alone won't reverse childhood obesity rates. She says that school-food reform has to do primarily with scoring political points. In other words, it is easier to attack the way government feeds children than the way their parents do.

"Food reformers need to make as strong a case for changing what kids eat outside school as what they do inside the cafeteria," she says. "Children are not 29 percent more likely to be obese because they eat school lunch, as that *American Heart Journal* study might seem to indicate. Instead, the children who eat school lunch—specifically, the ones who are most reliant on school meals—also are our poorest children: the ones without access to fresh produce in their neighborhoods, without parks and playgrounds to run around in, and, often, without parents who value good, healthy food."[9]

Kids eat plenty of fast food outside of school and have adjusted their appetites accordingly, points out Rhonda McCoy, Cabell County's school food service director. If you watched the *Food Revolution* program, you may remember Rhonda as the person in the middle of the school-lunch controversy in Huntington. I'll say this about Rhonda and most school officials: They care more about what kids eat than many parents do. After the first show, in which it appeared that Jamie Oliver was butting heads with Rhonda over our school lunch programs, the notes and emails that headed her way were a shame. Overzealous antagonists from around the country attacked Rhonda both professionally and personally—and regardless of how you feel about your local school lunch program, hurling expletives at the person who runs it is never acceptable.

It is also misguided. When it comes right down to it, administrators like Rhonda McCoy have very little to do with what food gets placed on local cafeteria tables. Besides, when you compare school lunches to what some kids bring from home, Rhonda is justified in feeling pretty good about the job she is doing. "One of the biggest problems school officials face is what parents send in their children's lunch boxes," Rhonda told me after the cameras left town. "Even affluent families pack processed entrees and junk food."

Despite the fiscal challenges of such a program, she advocates universal free lunches as a way to reduce the junk food coming into schools. "It's good to have fresh fruits and vegetables, and in many places they do have those options," she says. "It's getting better. But it all goes back to what parents are feeding children at home. The main thing parents need to do is model good behavior. If kids are eating fresh fruits and vegetables at home, then they're probably going to eat them at school. The biggest problem is that when we do serve fresh fruits and vegetables, the kids won't eat them. It doesn't do any good to make all these fresh meals if kids won't eat them because all they like is burgers and fries."

Rhonda is absolutely correct. One of the most frustrating things we encountered during the filming of the first *Food Revolution* was what we observed after Jamie instituted his fresh food menu at the local Central City Elementary. Some kids said they didn't like it, so they brought their own lunches from home, packed with sodium-rich processed foods, sodas loaded with sugar and caffeine, and Ziploc bags full of candy. Lunchbox after lunchbox, this was the norm! The very same parents sending these lunches were the ones complaining about Jamie providing healthier foods. I don't know how Rhonda dealt with it all.

Kids on the Move

When it comes to improving health at school, we can't focus on food to the exclusion of exercise. As Rhonda points out, parents everywhere should lobby their state officials for more recess. Sometimes regulations require so much instructional time that teachers are left with little or no flexibility. The result of these well-meaning but flawed policies has been a drastic reduction in school-time exercise. The CDC reports that in 1991, an average of 43 percent of high school students were taking gym class. By 2003, that number had dropped to 28 percent.[10] Here is where we can learn from Texas, whose state school board dropped mandatory gym classes in 1995 in an effort to strengthen academics. Six years later, they realized the error of their ways, reversed course, and started requiring more than two hours of weekly exercise to combat obesity.

"Right now the big push is to get kids involved in all the organized sports we can," says Rhonda's boss, Assistant Superintendent Mike O'Dell. "But when kids are involved in organized sports, a lot of their time is spent standing around while other kids are getting coached on technique. That may help the team when it comes to competing in athletic contests, but when you have free play, kids are running around constantly. If they're playing pick-up basketball, they're up and down the court all the time. When there's less structure, kids burn up more calories. The kids just need more time for recess."

I think the best things about free play, as opposed to organized sports, are that free play doesn't place time constraints on a family (you're not on someone else's schedule), and that it gives parents and kids an opportunity to exercise together. Parents at one Huntington school took this kind of insight to heart. Upset about having a substandard playground for more than 500 students, a group of parents at Kellogg Elementary talked with Principal Eugenia Damron. She told them there wasn't any money in the budget for playground improvements and suggested they try raising the funds. Raise the money they did!

Parents used their connections with a state senator to secure a $100,000 grant. Then, in about a year's time, the group raised another $70,000 and completed the job. The process included bake sales at grocery stores, donations from businesses and civic-minded individuals, and numerous small grants. Today, Kellogg is home to a jewel of a playground that includes a graveled, one-eighth mile walking track on the grounds, an adjoining (larger) track, and several fitness stations around its perimeter. Nearby are four basketball goals, jungle gyms, other exercise equipment, and a pair of orange towers, each with three platforms leading up to a series of slides.

Round 8 emphasized the importance of having a village to spread awareness of good health. No better example of a community coming together exists than this project. When they learned that installation of the playground equipment would cost an additional $30,000, parents organized a "community build." Workers included members of several trade unions, a National Guard unit, and other volunteers—more than three dozen businesses and community organizations played a role in the installation.

Dedicated in May 2010, the playground has made a huge difference in the school's outlook on physical fitness. Some students show up nearly an hour before classes to walk laps—including some who participate in a mileage program that offers rewards. Physical education teachers monitor their efforts. Adults got involved, too, forming a Couch-to-5K® program that initially drew 10 participants to workouts three times a week. As the playground neared its first anniversary, parent Melanie Shafer Adkins—a leader in the fundraising campaign—recruited volunteers to chaperone the site so children have proper supervision during playtimes.

Seeing the success of the program, the benefactor the fund-raising committee first approached was so impressed that he offered additional funds. That led to the start of "Tiger Pride" (named for the school's mascot) in January 2011. Held on Wednesday afternoons, this program requires parents to accompany their children instead of just dropping them off. During an hour-long session, participants take part in activities such as learning how to make healthy dishes, hearing a health talk from a local physician, and exercising with a group. Initial turnouts ranged from 80 to 120 pupils and parents. Thanks to the generosity of its benefactor, Tiger Pride had adequate funds to continue through the 2011-2012 school year. The program was barely a month old when Principal Eugenia from Kellogg Elementary received a request from another school in central West Virginia to visit and describe how Tiger Pride got started.

Citizen Action

These parents and administrators demonstrate how concerned citizens can take action to improve our schools' focus on health without waiting for higher authorities to act. No one ordered parents at Kellogg to go out and raise $170,000; they just put their heads together and devoted countless hours to the task. When April Hamilton wanted to bring a consulting firm to Charleston, she took the initiative to make that happen.

According to what I have seen from the outside looking in, it takes two things for a school to make a major change when it comes to creating a healthier environment: (1) a caring administrator like Eugenia Damron, and (2) some movin' and shakin' moms like Melanie Shafer Adkins and

April Hamilton. Parents may make their schools better places if they have that fire in their bellies, but they have to have cooperation from school officials. If you are a concerned mom or dedicated dad, go down to your kids' school and let the officials know you are there to help and have no desire to pack more responsibilities on their plates. I've never known a principal who wasn't overworked and underpaid. However, most principals want to see their schools get healthy, as long as they don't have to oversee the project or deal with any headaches. Just as we've seen at Kellogg Elementary, great things can happen when parents and administrators work together.

Although the school lunch scene is a complex situation where answers won't come easily, we should be encouraged. Parents can still take steps at the local level to improve their students' health—like Samantha Gotlib did. Samantha joined forces with another concerned mother, and in 2007 the pair founded a business that delivers organic lunches to thousands of students each month in the Orlando, Florida, area. There are similar grassroots initiatives elsewhere. All have goals of providing fresh, low-fat, healthy breakfasts and lunches to children. Some have even secured contracts to provide meals to public schools. All demonstrate how individuals with a vision can make a difference in their communities, regardless of what Uncle Sam does or does not do. The key, says Samantha, is raising parental awareness.

"I'm always amazed at how many parents don't realize the gravity of the situation," she says. "Our government is going into debt over healthcare, and yet they're sending people to the hospital, the doctor's office, the diabetes clinic. They're starting them off at six years old with what is going to cost them billions of dollars at the end of their lives. It makes no sense. Why not get all this processed stuff out of the lunch line and start serving kids fruits and vegetables? Then guess what happens 30 years from now? Healthcare costs will decrease."

Such a solution would seem like a no-brainer, but it's not. There are too many vested interests, too much money at stake, and too much resistance to change to easily loose the food chains binding America. As you are beginning to see, the food fight is much bigger than your home kitchen or school cafeteria. If we are going to win this boxing match, I believe God is going to raise up some people like the prophet Daniel—individuals who will go beyond the local school board and into the country's corridors of power. Ring the bell! It's time for Round 10.

Questions for Discussion

1. Have you encountered situations like April Hamilton did in trying to improve the quality of food at your school? What kind of food does your school have at its fundraisers? Without shouting or screaming, what can you do about it?

2. Regardless of the state or federal government, what changes can you make at your school to improve food quality?

3. Have you seen parents or other groups "storm the gates" at school board meetings to demand change? What can you learn from those situations?

4. What is a typical lunch at your children's (or grandchildren's) school? Does it consist of processed "reheat and serve" entrees, or real meat and an assortment of fruits and vegetables? How do you feel about that?

5. Do you think there are other parents in your community who care about their children's nutrition? If an action group doesn't already exist, what can you do to get one started?

6. How does the story of Kellogg Elementary's new playground inspire you? Are there steps you can take to improve recreational facilities in your area?

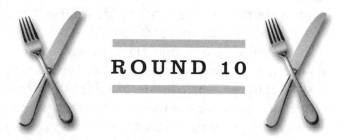

ROUND 10

The Politics of Food

At the conclusion of Jamie Oliver's filming in Huntington, it became clear to all of us that there was only so much our local educators could do for school lunches unless we had some help from the federal government. Consequently, the producers at ABC invited me to join Jamie in Washington, DC, to visit some national leaders who had considerable influence on school lunch policy. My naïve expectation was that our friendly government heads would welcome us with open arms and be thankful that we were trying to do something to help children in the "fattest city in America."

Boy, was I wrong.

Now, I am no stranger to Beltway politics. During my later teen years, my father was heavily involved in government issues as a United Mine Workers official. I tagged along on his business trips to DC whenever possible. I saw the frustration in his eyes when he attempted to pass mine safety regulations, only to be thwarted by interests that put miners' lives in harm's way. Looking back, if the legislation my father supported had passed, it is likely dozens of miners who were killed in recent West Virginia mining accidents would still be alive.

Twenty years later, I hoped for something better. Sadly, my return to our nation's capital was even more disappointing. You hear a lot about the caustic environment in Washington, and how it's worse than it has been in a long time. Until you are there, it is hard to understand how true that is. These days, there is very little spirit of cooperation. When it comes to things like school lunches and food for children in poverty, the partisanship amazes me.

The news isn't completely bad. There are some incredible people in Washington, DC, and I truly believe that many civic-minded individuals in the USDA and FDA have our best interests at heart. I also discovered some kindred spirits at the Pew Foundation. Although they are working at a nonprofit for relatively low pay, the people there are passionate about changing federal policies so that our children have access to proper nutrition and ultimately a chance to succeed in life.

On the other side of the coin was the inaptly named Center for Consumer Freedom (CCF). I left that office sick to my stomach. If I could rename it, I'd suggest that "Center for Hiding Information from Parents" or perhaps "Center for Nutritional Misinformation" would be more appropriate. Before we entered the building, Jamie warned me about what I was going to hear—but even with his admonition, I could not believe my ears. For 30 minutes, the CCF senior research analyst told us that fast food and sodas don't make people fat, that processed school lunches were just fine, and that the government was interfering too much with its support of our poorer children. He even claimed that the CDC report demonstrating the effects of poverty on obesity in West Virginia, and the press coverage that had surrounded it, made things sound worse than they really were.

"Oh," I asked, "you've been to West Virginia?"

"Yes," he replied. "Many times."

When I pressed him as to where, he informed me he had been to a few posh ski resorts near the Virginia border.

"Well," I replied, "if you ever want to drive past those ski resorts and come to my town, I'll introduce you to the *real* West Virginia." I explained that the majority of our families live on less than $25,000 a year, and that it was not uncommon for me to bury a 60-year-old heart attack victim or meet a mother whose child had been recently diagnosed with Type II diabetes. Somehow my personal experience only emboldened his resolve to explain why businesses and the industrial food chain had nothing to do with the plight of West Virginia's poor. He took another 10 minutes to explain why it is not our schools' responsibility to teach children about food, and why government statistics exaggerate our nation's health problems. After some time, it became clear to me that no matter what the evidence, he would criticize the source and never deal with the reality of our nation's obesity epidemic. In effect, he was saying, "Don't confuse me with facts; the food industry has no responsibility to the public on this issue."

As we were leaving, I noticed a number of cartoons on the wall, including one that made fun of Mothers Against Drunk Driving (MADD). You read that correctly—CCF was even antagonistic towards MADD! That's when it hit me. This place wasn't really a Center for Consumer Freedom. It was more akin to a powerful advocacy group for the very organizations that bear the greatest responsibility for our national health problems. After leaving DC and doing my own research, I found that this "nonprofit" organization arose via funding from the Phillip Morris Tobacco company[1] (around a $600,000 "donation") and had received contributions from other major benefactors like casinos, beer companies and slot machines. I thought, *Is there any vice that doesn't support this so-called freedom group?*

I share this story with you so you will understand this FACT: There are a number of powerful groups that profit greatly from our problems with food and drink. Just take a moment to consider that the food industry does more than a trillion dollars in sales annually; domestically, we spend over $800 billion a year on food and drink. At least 13 percent of our nation's gross national product is directly related to food consumption, and 17 percent of our labor force is involved in the food industry.[2] With all that money flying around, you'd better believe a lot of people want their piece of the action.

Please do not think for a minute that I am trying to act as an investigative reporter who has uncovered some clandestine conspiracy in Washington, DC. What I am about to share is well documented. Volumes of books and scholarly articles have been written on the subject, but for some reason the truth about our food industry has not made it to the masses. We continue to act in ignorance, having no clue just how unhealthy and corrupt our nation's food system has become.

In the next few pages, I'm barely going to touch the tip of the iceberg when it comes to food politics. You may be one who says, "I don't want the government to get involved in what I can and cannot eat." I agree! The problem is, the government has already become involved in our food choices, and their policies and subsidies are a large part of the problem. Instead of helping people get good information and proper nutrition, Uncle Sam is subsidizing the very industries that are killing us. To be honest, our national food culture is dirty, greedy, immoral and oppressive. As you will see, this is a moral issue. People are dying because of it. It is well past time for churches and concerned citizens to get involved.

Peas in a Pod

The similarities between Big Tobacco and the industrial food lobby are too striking to ignore. A generation ago, when science figured out how much damage tobacco-related products were doing to our national health, tobacco companies started flooding the information highway with their own "research," claiming that links between poor health and tobacco usage were inconclusive. It literally took acts of Congress to force those companies to tell the American people just how bad tobacco was for their health. Even then, people continued to smoke.

Today we face a marketing environment in which companies spend billions of dollars to confuse us about nutrition, leading the common, everyday citizen to throw up his or her hands and say, "I don't know what to believe." As a result, we keep on eating, just like our parents kept on smoking. Until we know for sure which foods actually kill us, most of us won't change our eating habits. Professor Marion Nestle, whom I mentioned previously, states, "Most of us believe that we choose foods for reasons of personal taste, convenience, and cost; we deny that we can be manipulated by advertising or other marketing practices."[3]

So while we keep right on eating, the food industry—like any other business—is constantly trying to figure out how to increase its profit margins. Of course, people are going to keep eating, but in order for food businesses to make *more* money than last year, the following will need to happen:

- Food production costs must decrease
- Food consumption/spending must increase
- Both of the above

It is easy to understand why food businesses want to find ways to influence us into consuming higher quantities of cheaply produced foods. The result will be the highest profit margins of all!

And that is exactly what has happened.

Cheap Food

Back in the 1970s, gas prices were going through the roof, and food prices were skyrocketing as well (sound familiar?). Farmers were going out of business, and families were struggling to feed their kids. In an effort to stem the tide, the United States government stepped in to help both groups.[4] The fastest and cheapest way to feed the most people the largest amount of food was with the multi-purpose *zea mays*—or, as it is more widely known: corn.

Traditional corn could be used not only as a side dish on a dinner plate, but also as popcorn, corn meal, corn bread, cornstarch, corn flakes, corn syrup, corn flour, corn chips and corn whiskey (just to name a few). In addition, agricultural scientists had discovered that corn could be manipulated in a number of ways to serve as the staple for an abundance of other cheap foods. Derivatives from chemically altered corn could serve as major in-gredients in baby food, beer, cereals, cheese spreads, mayonnaise, mustard and margarine, and as sugar substitutes in the form of sucrose, dextrose, glucose, and high-fructose corn syrup.

So Uncle Sam stepped in with subsidies and encouraged farmers to stop growing other veggies that cost a little more to produce and spoiled more quickly. In response, thousands left the fruit and vegetable business behind to focus on corn. The result was an overabundance of cheap corn flooding the market and driving down the costs of any food that used corn-based ingredients. In order to keep up with falling prices, even those who hadn't previously been using corn figured out ways to substitute it for other ingredients.

The problem was, the more farmers took advantage of Uncle Sam's subsidies, the more corn reserves *increased* and the more the cost of corn *decreased*. Suddenly, corn became so cheap to purchase that corn farmers weren't making enough profit on their crops to stay in business.[5] In order to help farmers, the government gave them more subsidies, but this fur-ther reduced the price of corn.

What could be done with all this cheap corn? How about making more high-fructose corn syrup and putting it in everything from soda to ketchup, salad dressings, muffins, peanut butter, jelly and . . . oh yeah, how about kids' cereals? I mean, what would be better than a bunch of husky, corn-fed football players? We all know that's how to fatten up those boys who are too slow to be running backs. (Unfortunately, it wasn't just ath-letes bulking up on all these corn derivatives.)

But there's still all this corn left over, and human beings can only eat so much of it. What shall we do? Enter the farm animal. Forget the fact that God made cows to eat grass. Nothing fattens up a steer like half a ton of corn! The same goes for pigs, chickens, and just about every other farm animal. Besides, it is a whole lot cheaper to buy 5 acres of land for 50 cows than 50 acres of land for 5 cows. You may have heard that God owns "the cattle on a thousand hills" (Ps. 50:10). Well, in modern America, Farmer Bob owns a thousand cattle, but he only has one hill! Just stick them all in a pen and feed them cheap corn. For Farmer Bob, that means no more bailing hay, maintaining miles of fencing, or chasing distant sounds of cowbells. Life is good.

For Betsy the cow, that means no more traipsing around the farmland in order to get food. Farmer Bob will bring her corn breakfast, and then all she has to do is lie around until it is time for corn dinner. Betsy will fatten up like never before, and her muscle will be marbled with fat like at no other time in history. Wow! What a deal. Farmer Bob couldn't be happier. It used to take three years of labor and expenses for a cow to reach the weight necessary to take it to slaughter. Now his cows grow so big so quickly that it only takes two years until Betsy is ready for the chopping block. That's a 33 percent faster turnaround for market, which means a lower cost of production. Consequently, the steaks that used to cost $12 a pound might have a little more fat in them, but Uncle Billy only has to pay $8 a pound at the local supermarket. Cheaper production. Cheaper food. Everybody wins, right?

For a while, it sure seemed that way. During the 1980s, our food system looked like a major success. I can remember my first visit to an all-you-can-eat pizza buffet—the experience set me back just $2.99. Dee and I both ordered the chopped steak and potato special for $1.99 each at the nearest Western Sizzler. Food was always at our beck and call, as fast-food restaurants and convenience stores were popping up on every corner. In the 1970s, there were approximately 70,000 fast-food shops. By 2001, there were 186,000.[6] Rich or poor, everybody had food and lots of it. God bless America!

Since this happened so quickly, I'm not sure if many people stopped to ask questions like, "Is it good for 50 cows to share one acre of space?" or "Is eating all I can consume a good thing?" Somewhere along the way, someone should have inquired, "How can a 16-ounce bag of corn chips that has been shipped halfway across the country in highly-decorated plastic and advertised on network TV be cheaper than 16 ounces of broccoli grown by a local farmer who spent nothing on packaging or advertising?"

Given a level playing field, I think fresh fruits and vegetables could give corn chips a run for their money, but they won't be able to if the government keeps subsidizing meat and grain production far more than fruits and vegetables. Only 9.8 percent of USDA subsidies go to fruits and veggies. The bulk of government assistance (72.7 percent) goes to grains (most of which goes to feed animals) and meat.[7]

Eat More and More and More

Once the industrial food complex had made major inroads in cutting the cost of food production (which meant a substantial increase in profits), the next step in tightening our food chains was to increase food consumption. Using their newfound income, companies who benefitted from government-subsidized meat and cheap corn (for instance, your favorite fast-food chain) began spending billions of dollars encouraging the masses to eat more and more of their cheap food. Around the turn of the century, the food industry was spending in excess of $33 billion annually trying to convince you that you needed more of whatever was making everyone else so fat and unhealthy.[8]

Don't get me wrong. I'm all about advertising a good deal. But something is wrong when 70 percent of advertising dollars go toward promoting heavily subsidized, unhealthy foods like candy, snacks, alcoholic beverages, soda and desserts. Meanwhile, just 2.2 percent of advertising encourages the purchase of fruits, vegetables, grains and beans.[9] Think about it: When's the last time you saw a commercial for plain old broccoli or spinach? Sweets, fats and salt—the "food group" with the highest profit margins—re-invest their earnings in commercials that bring them even greater profits.

Back in round five, I discussed how our bodies react to sweets, fats and salt. Something primal happens in the brain when we eat these substances. We literally become addicted to foods that contain high levels of them. Combine our instinctual need for them with the fact that they are some of the cheapest foods to produce and—whammo!—the companies peddling these goods get rich while America becomes the fattest nation in the history of the world. Is it any wonder said businesses spend so much on advertising? If they can get you to try their product, odds are you'll be hooked. People don't experience nervous shakes because they didn't have a green pepper for dessert, but bring out a piece of chocolate cake and watch them go wild.

So the cycle continues. We eat more sweets, fats and salt, and the companies that produce them make even more money. They then remind us through advertising that we need more of their product. The more they advertise, the more we eat. The more we eat, the more we crave. The more we crave, the more we buy. The more we buy, the more they profit. The more they profit, the more they advertise. This cycle repeats itself until the doctor tells you or your child, "You've got diabetes."

The sad part is that our politicians are not motivated to do anything about this. It's not like there are powerful lobbyists for carrots and green beans. Apple farmers aren't exactly making money hand over fist so they can compete with the campaign contributions of Big Corn, Fast Food, and various meat industries. Something has to change.

Food and Drugs/Drugs and Food

As we have seen, the industrial food chain has been wildly successful in increasing its profit margins at the expense of our national health and John Q. Taxpayer. While the powerful combination of EAT MORE/CHEAP FOOD has benefitted the food and drug industry, what about the ramifications for the rest of us? We already know that our waistlines have grown almost as quickly as their profit margins have. Could there be even more devastating outcomes as a result of our faulty policies and dirty politics? Let me suggest a couple: new strains of destructive bacteria and massive environmental damage.

Overdosing on Drugs

Last year, I picked up a prescription from our local pharmacy. I innocently asked the pharmacist (and our town's mayor), Rick Griffith, if I should finish the entire four-week prescription if I felt fine after two weeks. (Now let me tell you, I've preached some sermons before, but never in my wildest dreams did I think I'd get a lecture on pharmaceutical morality from a part-time politician.)

"Not only *should* you finish the prescription," he admonished, "but you owe it to your fellow man to do so."

"What?"

"Every time you take an antibiotic, the weakest strains of the bacteria are destroyed right away. Oftentimes this will lead to some symptomatic relief, but the stronger bacteria remain. The stronger bacteria will resist the effects of the antibiotic, and unless you finish off the infection entirely, you will only serve to make the resistant bacteria even stronger than before. In effect, you've inoculated the bacteria so that it becomes immune to the antibiotic it was exposed to, and it will take a more powerful antibiotic to destroy it in the future."

He had my attention.

"But it doesn't stop there," Rick continued. "You may be feeling well, but then you'll pass along that stronger bacteria to someone else and when they get sick, they might do the same thing you did with your prescription.

Each time bacteria is confronted with another antibiotic and it is not destroyed, the strain of bacteria will become even more resistant to antibiotics. Eventually, you end up with something like MRSA (Methicillin-resistant Staphylococcus Aureus), which is resistant to dozens of antibiotic treatments. Once that sets in, someone can get in big trouble. Hospitals are having a terrible time trying to treat people with these infections."

Rick said that pharmaceutical companies are encountering problems worldwide as they attempt to stay ahead of increasingly resistant strains of bacteria. The problem is compounded by the overuse of antibiotics, with many developing nations distributing them without prescriptions or medical advice. "If something doesn't change, someday these evolving bacteria are going to be so resistant to antibiotics, we're going to have to discover something else to fight infectious diseases that used to be cured by simple penicillin."

Then Rick said something that knocked me right out of my socks. "But you know, Steve, it's not just human consumption of antibiotics that are causing the problems. We're feeding so many drugs to animals right now, it's beyond belief."

I was in the middle of research for this round when he shared this insight. You would never think our problems with overeating and antibiotics were inter-related, but indeed they are. Nearly half of the antibiotics used in the United States are administered to animals, and this process is leading to antibiotic resistance in humans.[10]

The reason our farm animals need so many drugs is that the food industry, as I discussed earlier, finds it efficient to pack them into concentrated animal feeding operations (CAFOs) and stuff them full of corn. In these CAFOs, animals exist shoulder-to-shoulder at the corn trough, standing in their own manure and urine, spreading God only knows what diseases between them.[11] Enter E. coli, Mad Cow disease and other dangerous bacteria. The CDC estimates that more than 73,000 Americans are infected with E. coli each year, and at least 60 of those cases lead to death.[12]

Dress, Till and Keep

My maternal grandfather instilled in me a respect for the earth. He would quote the 1611 King James Bible and remind me that God's first commands to humankind were to dress, till and keep the earth. I never had any idea what that meant, but I knew it had something to do with gardening. Turns out, James Swain had become something of an environmentalist in his latter days. This change of heart came after he spent a lifetime pouring oil into the earth, throwing garbage along the creeks, and playing an integral role in an industry that ripped the tops off our mountains. All along, Grandpa knew what he was doing wasn't right, but he failed to make the connection that somehow he would be held accountable for his actions.

"I've not left this earth a better place," he sadly recollected as he weeded his mountaintop garden. "God gave us the task of taking care of HIS earth, and I don't think we're doing a very good job."

Around West Virginia, it is easy to see the damage done by the mining industry, but the food industry is much more subtle. My first realization of the effects of mass chicken production came a few years ago when I was fishing on the headwaters of the Potomac River (yes, *that* Potomac River—the one that flows right by our nation's capital).

Both my wife and I grew up fishing and camping on the South Branch of the Potomac, which runs through the eastern panhandle of West Virginia. George Washington was one of the first Europeans to explore these mountains; legend has it he caught a few fish there as well. From his time and through my college years, the South Branch was famous in the mid-Atlantic region for small-mouth bass. Even on a bad day, you could still catch a dozen fish.

My family returned to the river in 2008, and on the surface, everything looked the same. We were going to float downstream and catch some fish along the way. At the end of the day, we hadn't caught a thing. The water levels were a little low, but I had been there in lower levels than that. It didn't make sense. As soon as we came off the river, I went to visit an old friend who still had a place in the mountains. He had moved up in the world and become a top-ranking official in the federal government. After I had bemoaned my fishing experience for a few minutes, he stopped me before I could complain anymore.

"Ah, Stevie, it's not like it used to be," he lamented as he looked at the ground. "You probably would not have wanted to eat anything you caught anyway." Why? Because there are so many industrial chicken farms upstream that the nitrogen levels from their fecal matter have polluted the tributaries, and the fish are probably not safe to eat. In addition, he said the chickens are fed so many hormones that their urine has been shown to pass on those chemicals to the ground water in the area. "It's definitely caused some trouble to our ecosystem." (He went on to share that the locals know that when water levels get down, you don't even want to swim in the stream.)

Right now, there are thousands of chicken farms taking their toll on the streams of West Virginia and other states. Not only are these streams being polluted by animal waste, but also "testing has found evidence of antibiotics and antibiotic-resistant bacteria in many of the country's waterways."[13] Even if you don't eat the hormone-charged chicken meat, it is very possible your drinking water is affected by the more than 9 billion chickens that will be slaughtered this year alone.

Our meat-driven diet has led to an estimated 20 billion livestock in the world today,[14] and most of them will be killed this year. Think about that. That's three livestock for every one human being—a cow, a chicken and a pig for every single one of us on this earth.

Mining has been going on for hundreds of years, and the damage the industry has caused is severe, but if left undeterred, our current food system may well have effects on the environment that are more devastating than coal and oil combined. While it is difficult to comprehend, studies are telling us that global livestock production is doing more to produce greenhouse gases than all our planes, trains and automobiles combined![15] Not that the two categories are unconnected—our extra weight actually has a bearing on the amount of exhaust coming from combustible engines. According to the *American Journal of Preventive Medicine*, the extra 10 pounds the average American packed on in the last 10 years, taken collectively, caused the release of an extra 3.8 million tons of carbon dioxide through air travel.[16] Combine that with the effects of the extra weight we're towing around in our cars and trucks, and you're talking about an overwhelming amount of fossil fuel waste pouring into our earth—into the air, onto the land, and through our streams.

The mass production of animals is clearly driven by our perceived need to consume more and more meat. Simply stated, our planet cannot handle the demands we are placing on her resources. Not only is our appetite for more food destroying our bodies, but it is also destroying our planet. Because of our overwhelming need to fatten animals for excess meat, we have to chop down more forests so we can grow more corn. In turn, that gives us reduced access to antibiotics provided through nature. What does this do? As Rick Griffith told me, "It causes us to depend more on pharmaceutical companies to develop man-made, synthetic antibiotics, which are very, very costly." Health care costs go up—which is bad for us, but good for the pharmaceutical industry. After all, there's not much money for the medical industry if all they have to produce is that simple (and natural) penicillin.

The Incredible Hulk

I wish I could stop here, but the news gets worse. Knowing full well that tons of antibiotics are not enough to stop the spread of disease from animal meat to the humans who consume it, scientists came up with a wonderful idea. Instead of changing the way the industry produces meat or encouraging people to eat less meat, in 1997 the FDA approved the use of nuclear irradiation on our meats. Three years later, the USDA followed suit—and their approval of the practice included food to be used in school lunches.[17] I know you think I'm joking with you. I wish I were.

Have you ever had an X-ray? Unfortunately, I've had a number of them. So have our kids. When I was a child, I thought X-rays were cool. I once asked the attendant to zap me a couple more times so I could turn into the Incredible Hulk. My perspective has changed with age. Now I get concerned when I watch the radiologist run out of the room before he or she starts firing radiation through my body. Prolonged exposure to X-rays can cause serious damage to one's long-term health. The process of irradiating our meats—that is, the "deliberate exposure of food to nuclear radiation in order to kill pathogens"[18]—is the equivalent of more than 10 million chest X-rays.[19] I'm surprised my fast-food burger doesn't glow in the dark!

While the jury is still out on the overall safety of irradiation, studies have demonstrated chromosome damage in children after they were fed irradiated wheat for just six weeks. Dr. Don Colbert, author of *The Seven Pillars of Health*, reports, "When the children were taken off the diet, the condition went away."[20] A number of other studies suggest even more serious concerns.

Even if irradiation causes no immediate harm, as some organizations claim, it hasn't been around long enough to examine its long-term effects on the human body. My family is avoiding it at all costs. Thankfully, the USDA has required that irradiated food be marked with a Radura symbol—although some in the food industry are finding ways around letting you know that your food has been treated in this fashion. Always look for the following international symbol on packaged foods:

If you are eating at a restaurant, ask the manager if they serve irradiated foods. If he or she doesn't know the answer, eat somewhere else! Ask your local school nutritionist if they are serving such foods to your child—and whatever answer they give you, please get it in writing. I hate to advise that you go to such lengths, but until conclusive research demonstrates that this process is safe, I will remain skeptical—and Dee and I will keep our children as far from it as possible.

Even if irradiation is proven to be a viable option for destroying pathogens, the process still diminishes the nutrients of the food it has treated. Studies have demonstrated that irradiation destroys "up to 95 percent of vitamin A in chicken, 86 percent of vitamin B in oats, and 70 percent of vitamin C in fruit juices."[21] Yes, irradiating food usually kills what it's meant to kill, but it also negates the very reason God designed food for us to eat—nutrition.

Back to Eden

If I'm beginning to sound cynical, I apologize. It's just that when I look at the way God designed our food system and how it sustained us for thousands of years, and then I see what we have made it into today, I think, *No wonder we're in such a mess!* It is one thing to use our God-given talents to seek out more efficient and productive ways to steward the resources He's given us and quite another to throw the entire process into overdrive for the sake of unrelenting consumption.

What is God's system? Well, from the time of Noah to your grandpa's days on the farm, things were pretty much the same. God's sun and rain grew the grass, the grass fed the cows, the cows' manure fertilized the grass, and the system perpetuated itself. In addition, chickens ate parts of the cow manure, and what they excreted was an even better fertilizer for the crops (that is, unless you've got nine billion chickens). We humans were responsible for rotating those crops, making sure they were planted in land fertilized by our grazing livestock, and giving each section of the land a periodic rest (see Lev. 25:4). We ate the fresh crops as they came off the vine. Come Sunday dinner, we might have a little chicken and, on special occasions, beef. After dinner, we fed our slop to the pigs, and the meat from the pigs eventually fed us. With our energy from the farm-bred food, we took care of the offspring of the animals until they were able to take care of us. The system went on and on, just the way God designed it.

Well, maybe I should say, the way God allowed it.

Even the beautiful system I just described to you was not God's original design. No, in the beginning, humans didn't eat animals. (I'm going to type something now, but I want you to know it literally pains me to do so.) If we want to head back to a world where everyone gets food, where children don't go to bed hungry, and where greenhouse gasses aren't overwhelming our planet, *we have to eat less meat.* We have to heed the admonition of Proverbs 23:20: "Do not join those who drink too much wine or gorge themselves on meat."

There, I said it.

But it sure did hurt.

In no way, shape or form am I some kind of liberal elitist. I grew up in Cannelton "holler." I like to hunt, love to fish, and don't plan on stopping either of those activities any time soon. PETA is not likely to invite me to speak at its next annual convention. For goodness' sake, I went to the same high school as Zeke from Cabin Creek. (Though they may rescind my diploma for what I'm saying right now.)

However, deep down, I know that eating lots of meat is not good for me. As a follower of Christ, I cannot perpetuate our current food system by eating some kind of meat with every meal. I don't even need it once a day. I now know that producing one hamburger takes almost the same amount of resources as it takes to grow a dozen apples, a dozen tomatoes, or for that matter, a dozen ears of corn. Therefore, with all due respect to my friends at Christian-owned Chick-fil-A, I have decided to eat *less* chicken. Don't worry, my bovine friends—you and Mr. Pig are safer too. (But don't get too comfortable. God still gives me permission to occasionally eat meat, and I plan to exercise that freedom!)

While one can argue the pros and cons of including meat in one's diet, it is difficult to argue the innate wisdom of our traditional, farm-based food system. Compare that system to the modern industrial food complex. There is not much of a cycle here, and ultimately the process culminates in a one-way, dead-end street.

Why do I say that? We mass produce genetically altered corn with as many artificial fertilizers as possible. We never give the land any rest, thus robbing it of most nutrients, which eventually forces us to leave the useless land behind. We then chop down more forests—which, as we all know, give us oxygen and remove carbon dioxide from our atmosphere. We drive combustible engines hundreds of miles to ship this corn to chemical factories so they can make it into sugars, syrups, oils and starches that are manipulated even more to create the food that fattens us and hardens our arteries. What's left over (60 percent of all corn grown), we send to concentrated animal feeding operations, which are breeding grounds for *E. coli* and many other diseases. We bulk up the animals with genetically altered corn so we can get them to market more quickly. Their meat has much more fat than that of grass-fed animals, because corn has a way of doing that to animals too, and of course this fat-laden meat makes the humans who consume it all the fatter as well. But what about the diseases in the meat? Don't worry about that—we'll just nuke them and feed what's left to our children.

Makes sense to me.

As I stated earlier, I don't expect our government to fix this problem any time soon. The system I just described is making too much money for too many people. As Michael Pollan describes in *The Omnivore's Dilemma*, King Corn will continue to drive the industrial food complex, because in our economy the growing of corn supports the larger economy—which includes, but is not limited to, "the chemical and biotech industries, the oil industry, Detroit, pharmaceuticals (without which they couldn't keep animals healthy in CAFOs), agribusiness, and the balance of trade. Growing corn helps drive the very industrial complex that drives it. No wonder the government subsidizes it so lavishly."[22]

Vote with Your Fork

If you are like me, sometimes you just want to put your head back in the sand and forget it. It is easy to throw up our hands and continue with the status quo. That is the reason for so many conflicting messages out there. I believe the food industry *wants* us to feel overwhelmed and confused. This "overwhelm them and confuse them" strategy kept Big Tobacco on the scene long after it should have been extinct. Though our fast-food "friends" know they've been exposed, they're going to hang on for as long as they can and make as much money as they can.

That's where you can make a difference.

Most of us don't have inside connections to our legislators, but all of us can hit the EAT MORE/CHEAP FOOD groups where it hurts: in the wallet. Unlike our bureaucratic government, food and retail companies respond quickly to consumer demand. If they don't, they will go out of business. If we don't buy their product, they will quit producing it.

You have the power to educate yourself about food and where it comes from, and to buy healthy foods. Every dollar is a vote. In the same way, if you buy unhealthy fast food, you vote to perpetuate the problem. Your choices are bigger than you. That's right—if you take your kids to the nearest fast-food outlet and order unhealthy foods, that is a vote to fatten up the kids of America. But if you buy fresh produce from local farmers, that is a vote to break the industrial food chain—and it's another step toward winning the food fight. Here's the really good news. You don't just get to vote one time. You vote every single time you go to the grocery store. You vote every time you order something off a menu. You vote by packing a lunch for your kids if your school is using irradiated meats. Vote, vote, vote!

For those who do have connections in our government (and my prayer is that God will get this book into the hands of people who can make a difference), here are some ideas for legislation that I, and many others, believe could make an incredible impact on our nation's future.[23] As stated before, I don't think government needs to get involved in everything, but since they helped get us into this problem, they have an obligation to help get us out of it.

1. *Education.* Every child in our school systems needs to be taught about food and where it comes from. It is no accident that where educational levels are the highest, obesity levels are the lowest. Sadly, the reverse is also true. Our least-educated states (like my good old West Virginia) are also the most obese. The great common denominator in America is education. We have to give our kids a chance.

2. *Labeling.* Give concerned parents the information they need to make good choices. Require the food industry to list all ingredients on packaging. If any ingredient in any food has been

through the irradiation process, parents need to know. Right now, companies don't have to label food as irradiated if only some of the ingredients have been nuked.

3. *Restaurant listings.* I don't want to hurt small businesses, but large chains should provide nutritional information for each item on the menu. Exactly how much sugar, fat and salt are in this meal? Again, parents need to know.

4. *Soda tax.* Just like cigarettes, soda is causing a health care crisis in this country. It is not fair to those of us who have decided to take care of our bodies to make us pay higher taxes for increased health care programs. Tobacco companies were forced to pay into our system for all the damage they have done to our national health. It is high time we expected soda companies to do the same.

5. *Subsidize fresh fruits and vegetables.* This seems like a no-brainer to me. Reduce the subsidies given to grains and meats (currently 73 percent of the total budget) and increase amounts for fruits and vegetables (currently only 9.8 percent).[24] We have to get the cost of fresh produce down to more affordable prices so that lower-income families and individuals have healthy food options. If you don't like government involvement, fine. Cut *all* subsidies and let the free market work it out. That would be better than our current system.

Calling for Help

As I have said throughout this book, we cannot separate the physical from the spiritual or the secular from the eternal. There are greater forces involved in this food fight than governmental bureaucrats and business moguls. When we see children diagnosed with fatal diseases, thousands of Americans hospitalized annually with food-borne illnesses, and our planet being destroyed by the same system that sickens its inhabitants, the players involved are much larger than mortal men. I'm not one to blame all problems on a cartoonish devil with a pitchfork, but if you believe the words of Scripture, you must accept that some of the world's philosophies are driven by dark spiritual forces (see Eph. 6:10-20). Even people who don't believe in God realize this food fight is a battle between good and evil. Therefore, we should not wage this battle ourselves. That is why I believe the next round holds the key to winning this match.

Questions for Discussion

1. Does it surprise you that there are groups in Washington, DC, whose major role is to support the profits and interests of the food industry? Why or why not?
2. What similarities do you see between the tobacco companies and our food system? How can we implement the strategies used against Big Tobacco to bring about nutritional changes on a nationwide basis?
3. Of all the behind-the-scenes industry information shared in this round, what piece was the most troubling to you? Why?
4. Have you ever wondered why entire bags of greasy, processed, chemical-laden chips are cheaper than plain, fresh vegetables? How did this situation come to be?
5. In what ways is our love affair with meat so detrimental to our health and environment?
6. How will your nutritional choices change as a result of what you have just read?
7. How can we utilize both the power of legislation AND the free-market system to improve the way we do food economics?

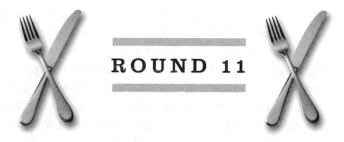

ROUND 11

Life in the
Fast(ing) Lane

I have an incredible knack for choosing the slow line at the grocery store. No matter what time of day I go or which register I choose, invariably I get stuck behind someone who argues with the cashier, asks for a price check, or sends their kid back to retrieve a gallon of milk. It drives me crazy. My blood pressure rises every time I get stuck in a line that is supposed to be moving, but turns into the slow lane. It is no different on the interstate. Please don't ask me to drive on the right side. I love zooming along in the high-occupancy-vehicle lane while others crawl through rush hour traffic. I like to keep moving—fast.

If you are like me, when you see something that needs to be accomplished, you want it done yesterday. Likewise, if your eyes have been opened to the food chains that bind your life and the lives of friends and family members, I'm sure you want to make progress in the food fight *right now*. With God's help, I believe that together we can make a difference and *some* changes can take place quickly. Yet, as our community edges toward better health, I am reminded that sometimes a slower method is superior.

I love the biblical account of how Jesus sent His disciples out to help people with their physical needs. The disciples' initial success turned to frustration when they encountered a young boy experiencing seizures. They repeatedly tried to heal him, but to no avail. After Jesus arrived and surveyed the situation, He immediately healed the child. The disciples were confused. They had helped heal dozens of people—why not this boy? I can just see Jesus pulling those young men over to the side and softly reminding them, "But this kind does not go out except by prayer and fasting" (Matt. 17:21, *NASB*).

Friends, some things in life only need a quick decision to resolve the problem. Other things we deal with take considerable work and determination, but we can eventually make them better by ourselves. However, occasionally—like the disciples—we encounter a problem that we cannot fix. As in the tale of Humpty Dumpty, "all the king's horses and all the king's men" can't put things back together again. In such cases, I turn to a variation on Christ's words: "This can only be fixed by fasting and prayer." As a pastor, I wish I could tell you I am enthusiastic about fasting and prayer. Unfortunately, I cannot. Too often I want the *fast* track more than I want the *fasting* track.

On the fast track, I can move under my own power. Paved with a little more education, it is for those who think they have all the answers. These people will run you over if you get in their way. I have to admit it, I like the fast track, and I tend to run with other fast-track people.

The *fasting* track is much slower. It keeps us focused on our dependence on God and others. It is nowhere near as dramatic as a six-week reality TV series. Yet the fasting track is where life's biggest problems get solved. It is the road less traveled by man but most traveled by God. As I contemplate the food fight facing this nation, I see a problem with roots much deeper than a few pieces of legislation can resolve. If Jesus were among us in bodily form today, I believe He would give us the same advice: "This kind can only come out through prayer and fasting."[1]

You may not be a religious person. However, before just skipping on to the next round, will you give this one a chance? For thousands of years, people have found answers through fasting. I don't want us to be so set in our "here and now" ways that we cannot explore an avenue of liberation that may be the most freeing of all. The discipline of this practice is not just for ascetic monks in the foothills of the Himalayan Mountains.

Feast or Famine?

Traveling to foreign countries gives one a perspective that cannot be gained from remaining in the comforts of home. I don't mean stopping at resorts that cater to the desires of rich Americans. I'm referring to immersing oneself in a culture—sleeping where the people sleep, playing where they play, working like they work, and eating what they eat. One thing I have learned from overseas travel is that sometimes varying cultural values are subtle; other times, they hit you square in the face.

In every society, people have blind spots they struggle to recognize. They become so conditioned by their culture that they can't see what is painstakingly obvious to others. Such was the case when some of our friends from the Zambian International Theological College came to West Virginia. After I had spent nearly a month sharing life with fellow believers in Zimbabwe, Zambia, South Africa and Swaziland, I couldn't wait to give some of my brothers the opportunity to visit us in the United States. Our church raised the money to bring a few of them to a statewide conference so they could share about their educational ministries and tell us about the plight of orphans left behind by the AIDS epidemic.

When they arrived, we wanted to give our guests the best we had to offer. A few families hosted them; everyone made sure they didn't miss a meal. Two weeks into their visit, one of the pastors pulled me to the side and said, "Pastor Steve, I have a question for you. It seems as though in America every meal is a feast. You people don't eat; you feast. I have never seen so much food."

Ouch. Granted, I was aware of our people's problematic eating habits. Still, I thought these gentlemen would enjoy the opportunity to sample America's varieties and quantities of foods. After all, it was only for a few weeks. Surprisingly, though, it wasn't our gluttonous practices that bothered my friend most deeply. His next question socked me between the spiritual eyes: "We've been here two weeks, and we eat three or four times every day. When do you take the time to fast?"

He didn't have to say another word. With a humbled spirit, I admitted that we Americans don't fast much. I could not name one church in West Virginia that fasted on a regular basis. As part of my research for this book, I looked for studies on the percentage of Americans and/or Christians who fast for ANY reason—spiritual, medical, physical or otherwise. I cannot begin to tell you how difficult it was to find any such information. Next time you're in a Christian bookstore, take a look around you. Signs everywhere point you in the direction of sections on basic theology, church growth, family living and personal success. For a fun experiment, try asking someone at the front desk to direct you to books dedicated to the topic of fasting. I've done this a few times, and it's a real blast. While most workers have been congenial, some of the comments I have received are:

- "Fasting? What's that?"
- "You mean like not eating?"
- (After a 10-minute search) "I'm sorry; I can't find it. I remember seeing one of those about a year ago."
- My favorite: "Isn't that a Muslim thing? We don't carry that stuff here."

This is not to say that books on fasting are not available. Dr. Elmer Towns of Liberty University has written extensively on the subject. A quick search on Amazon.com yields hundreds of titles. However, many people in the pews don't care. "Fasting is for super-Christians," one parishioner told me. "I'll save that for when I'm really in trouble." Such ambivalence didn't exist in biblical times. Though it had become a source of pride for some, many practiced fasting twice a week (see Luke 18:12). Abstaining from food was as normal as things like praying and giving to the needy. Consider these verses from Matthew 6:

> So *when* you give to the needy, do not announce it with trumpets. . . . But *when* you give to the needy, do not let your left hand know what your right hand is doing, so that your giving may be in secret. . . . And *when* you pray, do not be like the hypocrites, for they love to pray standing in the synagogues and on the street corners to be seen by men. . . . But *when* you pray, go into your room, close the door and pray to your Father, who is unseen. . . . *When* you fast, do not look somber as the hypocrites do, for they disfigure their faces to show men they are fasting. I tell you the truth, they have received their reward in full. But *when* you fast, put oil on your head and wash your face (vv. 2-6,16-17, emphasis added).

Notice that Jesus did not say "if" you give or "if" you pray or "if" you fast. Just as He assumed His followers would pray and give to the needy, He assumed they would fast. Every church prays during their worship services, and they usually take an offering. But what happened to fasting? Dr. Towns recalls that he once had someone tell him he needed to write on the topic because "no one had written a bestselling book on fasting in 100 years."[2]

One cannot help connecting the spiritual dots between our national obsession with food and our lack of fasting. Food has such a stronghold on the American church that even its leaders don't discipline themselves when it comes to abstaining for spiritual reasons. Simply stated, we don't fast because we are addicted to physical pleasures.

As I mentioned before, there are a number of in-depth books on fasting, and I encourage you to expand your knowledge of the discipline beyond what I address in this brief excursion. However, for the remainder of this round, I will review fasting's basics, its benefits, and why learning this discipline may hold the key to winning the food fight.

Fasting 101

Since there is considerable confusion over the idea, it may be best to start with a working definition. Fasting is voluntary abstinence from eating all or certain foods for one or more specific purposes. There doesn't seem to be a specific time frame associated with fasting. The Bible contains examples ranging from a few hours to 40 days. Sometimes people abstained from all food and drink; other times they gave up just food, or certain kinds of food and drink. There are so many different examples that I'm led to believe that the Bible doesn't prescribe a particular type.

No matter what kind you choose, fasting should not be taken as a recipe for righteousness or a kind of magical incantation by which we can impress God or convince Him to grant our wishes. He is not manipulated through human effort. In fact, I believe that the opposite is true: Fasting is God's way of transforming us. Much like prayer, fasting is a mechanism God uses to change us into the people He wants us to be. He doesn't ask us to fast for His sake, but for ours.

Though I could give you a top 10 list of reasons to fast, I worry that you would interpret the first as the most important. Fasting doesn't work like that. It is not about the parts, but the whole. As we learn to fast, we gain spiritual, mental, emotional and physical benefits. For example, one of my good friends fasted from all food and drink (other than water) for nearly 40 days. After a number of days, his mind became sharper than at any previous time in his life. Though looking for spiritual enlightenment, he achieved a mental breakthrough. In particular, cutting off his intake of sugar improved his memory and helped him communicate more clearly.

The results didn't stop there. After three weeks, people asked what he was doing to lose weight. Though this was not his intent, he lost more than 40 pounds over the course of a month. Physically, he felt better than he had in years. Spiritually, he became more keenly aware of the barrage of food advertisements he encountered during an average day. One morning, he decided to take note of the images that confronted him throughout the day—but by afternoon, he stopped counting at 150. *No wonder I struggle so much with my diet*, he thought. *Everywhere I turn, somebody is trying to get me to buy their food product.*

My friend's experience taught me that fasting has a plethora of benefits, all of which are important. Some may emphasize one benefit over another, but this falls back into our dualistic habit of elevating one aspect of who we are over the other aspects. If you get no other message from this book, please appreciate this: You cannot separate who you are spiritually from who you are mentally or physically. In the pages that follow, I will discuss fasting's physical, mental, emotional and spiritual benefits individually, but please keep in mind that the goal is to improve as a whole person. Ultimately, my prayer is that, by fasting, you will find breakthroughs in all areas of life.

Physical Benefits

Obviously, if you go without food on any extended basis, you *will* lose weight. At the same time, for someone struggling with his or her physical health, I would never recommend abstaining from food for long periods of time. In fact, I would never recommend that anyone begin fasting without first consulting a physician. Nevertheless, it stands to reason that we will likely eliminate some of our physical problems if we stop consuming the foods that contribute to them. In his bestselling book *The Maker's Diet*, Dr. Jordan Rubin describes how the body often heals itself when it is not busy digesting food. Rubin explains that the body needs time to purge itself from various toxins and other substances to which we expose our stomachs, livers and kidneys daily. Because we eat so much and so often, we keep our organs in virtual overdrive.

One study examined the progress of 156 patients who were dealing with a number of physical illnesses, including ulcers, heart disease, sinusitis, insomnia, asthma and even cancer. After participating in fasts spanning between 5 and 55 days, the patients demonstrated the following results:

- 113 completely recovered
- 31 partially recovered
- 12 were not helped
- 92 percent improved or totally recovered[3]

This and similar studies are difficult to ignore. From what I have observed, research indicates that with regard to such conditions as obesity, intestinal problems, arthritis and even diabetes, the solution may be found in fasting alone. (I must encourage you again, before trying a fast of any substantial duration, to consult your doctor. If your body is not used to fasting, going off food cold turkey may not be the best way to begin.

Remember that taking fasting to extremes—doing it too often or using laxatives and other faddish methods—may *cause* physical problems instead of solving them.)

While there is much more to be said about the physical benefits of fasting, for the purposes of this review I will simply say that even if there were no spiritual, mental or emotional benefits to the practice, it would still be worth your time. If God chose to rest after six days of creation, surely your digestive system could use a periodic rest as well.

The Sabbath principle—the need for a time of rest—is pervasive throughout the Scriptures. Ultimately, our problem with food is a result of a nonstop society that pushes our children to produce more, our animals to produce more, our land to produce more, and our digestive systems to produce more. The Sabbath principle is God's way of reminding us that our worth is not found in what we produce. We have value because we belong to our Creator—and that same Creator is exclaiming to us, "Give things a rest!"

Mental Benefits

Every person I interviewed about fasting told me that the effect on their mental capabilities was one of the most striking aspects of their experience. I have found the same to be true in my own life. However, I do not want you to believe that the only kind of fasting that sharpens your thinking skills involves total abstinence from food. Another pastor at our church, Joe Dorsey, practiced a fruit-and-vegetable diet he called the "Daniel Fast" (see Round 4). For nearly three weeks, in addition to meat, Joe and his wife, Nancy, also eliminated caffeine and sugar from their diet, to the point that Nancy experienced severe withdrawal headaches. "For the first few days, we were both miserable," says Joe. "I was grouchy, and Nancy just stayed in bed. We began to wonder if we had bitten off more than we could chew." However, by persevering they discovered how their unhealthy diet had impeded their lives. "I don't know that I have ever thought so clearly," Joe says. "There's really no way to describe it. We thought better, prayed better and ate better, but most importantly, we learned to discipline ourselves in the area of food."

Joe's experience is not unique. Once you outlast the initial headaches that usually accompany fasting, you are likely to achieve mental and spiritual peace. Initially, our bodies crave the toxic foods they are used to having, but eventually the clouds open, and a sense of accomplishment takes precedence. The symbiotic relationship between mind, body and spirit acquires a whole new meaning.

Spiritual and Emotional Benefits

I enjoyed my first experience with fasting at the age of 26. Sadly, during my first 18 years of Christian life, including 8 as a youth pastor and 4 in seminary, I had never been seriously challenged to engage in fasting. Even then, I only tried it because I wanted to teach our youth group what it felt like to be hungry. I reasoned that going 30 hours without food would help them empathize with the poor and inspire them to raise more money for World Vision (a leading charity that deals with poverty in developing nations).

A dozen high school students volunteered to participate. I didn't trust them to stick with their commitment, so I called for a lock-in at the church. After a snack at 11:59 PM on a Friday, we wouldn't eat again until breakfast (the true meaning of *break-fast*) on Sunday morning. When we went to sleep at 2 AM, everyone seemed to be doing fine. By 10 AM Saturday, everyone was awake and drama had erupted. One girl got mad at another over a curling iron, two guys got into a fight during a basketball game, and around noon one girl just started crying (I still don't know why). At that point, one teen called his mother to come get him, saying he couldn't handle the pressure.

Pressure? We had skipped one meal and he couldn't handle the *pressure?* As soon as he left, two other kids called home. Suddenly I had a grandmother on the phone, chewing me out for expecting kids to go without food *for one whole day.* I had to admit, this was affecting all of us emotionally, myself included. Though amazed by our spiritual weakness, at that moment I experienced a deep spiritual insight: *No wonder teenagers struggle with sex, drugs and alcohol. They are controlled mentally and emotionally by the desires of their flesh.*

Adults are no different. Until we learn to discipline our desires, we will not overcome our addiction to food. Like no other exercise, fasting teaches us that discipline—and if we can control our eating habits, we will likely be able to control other physical choices. This lesson is inherent in the story of Jesus in the Garden of Gethsemane (see Matt. 26). Facing imminent betrayal, Jesus asked His disciples to stay up late to pray with Him. After leaving for a short while (to spend time in prayer

Himself), Jesus returned and found them asleep. He knew they cared and wanted to be there for Him, but their need for sleep overcame that desire. Within this context, Jesus offered His famous comment: "The spirit indeed is willing, but the flesh is weak" (Matt. 26:41, *KJV*).

When it comes to nutritional choices, there is no other statement that better sums up our existence. I find that most people want to eat well, so they will feel good and look good, but their flesh overcomes that desire. To me, the most beneficial aspect of fasting is this: It has taught me how to say "no" to my flesh and "yes" to God. It has taught me that man does not live by bread alone (see Matt. 4:4), and that food is not my master (nor, for that matter, is any other interest that may compete with God's will for my life). As God said to Cain, "Sin . . . desires to have you, but you must master it" (Gen. 4:7).

As I have learned to discipline my flesh, it amazes me how much my relationship with God has improved, affecting other areas of my life. Paul urges, "Live by the Spirit and you will not carry out the desires of the flesh. For the flesh has desires that are opposed to the Spirit, and the Spirit has desires that are opposed to the flesh, for these are in opposition to each other, so that you cannot do what you want" (Gal. 5:16-17, *NET*). Through these words, you can see the effect dualism had on Paul's teaching. We know that the body is not evil, and that it is a gift from God. Still, there is something about the desires of the "flesh." What is it about our fleshly needs that cause us to chase after the things of the here-and-now as opposed to the greater, eternal good? The desire to feed and take care of our bodies is not sinful. However, if not kept in check, it can serve as a distraction. If we choose to indulge in distractions to the detriment of our overall good, *that* is a sin.

If the desire to please the flesh were a sin, then Jesus Himself would have been a sinner (which, of course, He was not). His victory over temptations of the flesh demonstrated His sinless nature. Consider His temptation in the desert (see Matt. 4). The Bible says that after fasting for 40 days and nights, He was hungry—which has to be the greatest understatement in Scripture. Despite this extreme hunger, Jesus maintained control of His physical urges. Although He had the ability to turn a stone into a piece of bread, He refused. It was not that eating would have been evil, but rather that losing the ability to control His actions would not reflect the fruit of self-control (see Gal. 5:23).

This story offers us a great lesson. It was not a full belly that prepared Jesus to deal with temptation, but an empty one. Indulging the flesh does not control it. Indulgence is the means by which the flesh controls us.

When Jesus resisted His hunger for 40 days, it prepared Him to face the devil. That is the beauty of fasting: It reveals the things that control us or want to control us.

The Emancipation Proclamation

Unless they fast, most people never realize how much they are enslaved to their cravings. This is not to say that appetites are a bad thing. God gave us physical pleasures to enjoy, but these pleasures become spiritually damaging when we allow them to control us. Paul states, " 'Everything is permissible for me'—but not everything is beneficial. 'Everything is permissible for me'—but I will not be mastered by anything" (1 Cor. 6:12). That begs the question: Are you mastering your food, or is food mastering you?

God made us to desire physical and spiritual pleasures. Yet, when our natural cravings begin to master us, we worship the gifts instead of the One who gives them. The apple is never greater than the One who grew the apple tree. As Adam and Eve learned through sweat and tears, choosing the created thing over the Creator is the essence of idolatry. If we are honest, many of us will admit that at times we worship at the feet of our refrigerators. Fasting teaches us to desire the Creator more than His creation. It is only when we give our total selves to God that we are truly set free (see Romans 6 and 8).

Ultimately, God's goal for your life is that you learn to desire Him more than you desire the things of this world. Since fasting is an integral part of that process, I am convinced that the Church will never know God's power until we practice it. Furthermore, as I learned from personal observation, until we get our eating habits under control, we are not going to be able to fast. Asking those teens to fast for 30 hours was like asking them to jump over the moon. They didn't have the skills or the strength required. So here we have a chicken-or-the-egg situation. If we want to win the food fight, we need to practice the discipline of fasting. Yet, we don't have the wherewithal to stick to our commitments. Where do we start? We begin by learning to be hungry.

Developing a Greater Hunger

The Bible is filled with metaphors. The bride-and-groom metaphor in Ephesians 5 describes Christ's love for His people. Hosea married the prostitute

Gomer as a metaphor for God's unending love for us, even when we chase after other gods. Hunger is a metaphor for things that drive us. If a baseball player is described as "hungry" for a championship, that means he has a drive to win. A young woman who is "hungry for affection" deeply desires a relationship with someone who will care for her.

Can you say you have a hunger for God? King David once proclaimed, "My soul yearns, even faints, for the courts of the LORD; my heart and my flesh cry out for the living God" (Ps. 84:2). In another psalm, David used the metaphor of thirst when he cried out, "As the deer pants for streams of water, so my soul pants for you, O God. My soul thirsts for God, for the living God. When can I go and meet with God?" (Ps. 42:1-2). We can learn a great lesson from the psalmist. More than anything else—more than our desire for food after a hard day's work or a drink after a long run—something in our souls should yearn to know the God who loves us.

When we tap into that kind of powerful relationship, it is more soothing than the feeling we get from that first bite of food or that first sip of cold, crisp water. Fasting makes these metaphors explode in your consciousness, pointing you to a realization of your greatest need. As I have developed this practice (and I have a long way to go), I have discovered that abstaining from food gives me a desire to do other things that do not come naturally. When I fast, I often find myself:

- Discovering overlooked sins. Fasting quickens my spirit, and the "little" things that once escaped my attention come to the forefront of my consciousness. Fasting exposes my personal shortcomings, gives me the opportunity to confess those faults to God, and allows me the opportunity to grow in my faith.

- Tuning in my spiritual radar to God's will. When I find myself at a spiritual crossroads or facing a crucial decision, fasting improves my ability to hear God's Spirit. When I need to intensely seek God's guidance, fasting is the key to finding direction (see Judg. 20:22-28; Ezra 8:23; Neh. 1:4; Dan. 9:3; Acts 13:3; 14:23).

- Gaining opportunities to display spiritual fruit. Many times, we ask God to give us patience without realizing that He does so by placing us in situations where we have to exercise patience. If we ask for courage, God puts us in a position where we have to demonstrate courage. When I pray for God to give me self-control, He has a way of setting me down in a restaurant with 100 dessert choices. Fasting prepares me for these situations that build my character so I can face the next challenge God has for me.

- Becoming more dependent on God. If nothing else, fasting shows me my weaknesses. In such times, I am forced to rely on God, just as Jesus did when tempted in the desert. When God allows us to experience hard times or causes us to hunger, it is His way of teaching us that we do not live on bread alone, but by every word that proceeds from His mouth (see Deut. 8:2-3).

- Refusing to be satisfied with temporary pleasures. Why do we get so bent out of shape over things that have no eternal value? In the winter of 2011, I wrecked my truck. The repairs cost nearly $2,000. Even worse, I had to rob my vacation fund to pay the bill. I had worked long and hard to earn that money, and because of a patch of ice, it vanished in an instant. I couldn't believe a fender bender cost me a week's vacation. I fretted and fumed. (I even got mad at God for allowing the accident to happen!) Dealing with frustration, I fasted and prayed, hoping $2,000 would drop out of the sky. Instead, within a few hours, God gave me a new perspective. I didn't need $2,000, a truck or a vacation. I just wanted God to be pleased with His servant, Steve.

The most temporary thing this world has to offer is the meal set before us. Yet, even when armed with the knowledge that whatever we eat will be digested and excreted in a short time, we can value food so much that we are willing to pay 50, 75 or even 100 dollars for that "one great meal." By skipping a meal here and there, and eating out less frequently, we can say "no" to temporary pleasures and "yes" to this next type of fast—the type God says He really wants to see.

The Fast that Matters

The Bible is full of stories of hypocrites and blowhards. In Christ's day, religious folk represented our Savior's number-one enemy—especially the leaders who loved power, drew the equivalent of million-dollar salaries from the contributions of those of modest means, and looked for ways to use God's name for self-promotion. Jesus said the hottest spots in hell are reserved for such people (see Luke 20:47). Sadly, we can be sure that modern-day churches still contain such Pharisees.

One of my favorite chapters in the Bible is Isaiah 58. Directed specifically toward religious people, including those who fasted, God commanded His prophet to shout these words. He had grown tired of His children waltzing off to weekly worship services, giving a few cents to the priest, and expecting showers of blessings. They had full bellies, nice houses, and peace and security at home, but they ignored those who were less fortunate. Sure, they skipped a meal here and there, but they were missing what James (in James 1:27) called the essence of true religion:

> Is not this the kind of fasting I have chosen: to loose the chains of injustice and untie the cords of the yoke, to set the oppressed free and break every yoke? Is it not to share your food with the hungry and to provide the poor wanderer with shelter—when you see the naked, to clothe him, and not to turn away from your own flesh and blood? Then your light will break forth like the dawn, and your healing will quickly appear; then your righteousness will go before you, and the glory of the LORD will be your rear guard. Then you will call, and the LORD will answer; you will cry for help, and he will say: Here am I (Isa. 58:6-9).

I could preach a month of sermons from this one chapter, but here I just want to highlight a few points. Do you see the kind of fast God desires—the kind that gets His attention and tells Him we are serious about depending on Him? This fast can be summarized as abstaining from any behavior that inhibits us from:

• Stopping injustice
• Freeing the oppressed
• Feeding the hungry
• Giving shelter to the homeless
• Clothing the needy

Do you want God's help with winning the food fight? Do you want Him to show up and say, "Here am I"? A good way to start is by breaking the chains of injustice. Do you think Jesus is concerned about race or nationality when a young girl needs a meal or healthcare? How would Jesus help a young boy whose parents want to get him out of a failing school, but there aren't enough spots in the school across the tracks? Expand your horizons a little and think about the 5 million children worldwide who died in 2010 because they didn't have enough food.[4] It amazes me that some of God's children in the United States are going to die prematurely due to OVEReating, while around the world children are dying due to UNDEReating. What a cruel, inhumane joke by the forces of greed and gluttony!

Now, you may be saying, "I know this is a problem, but what can I do to help? It's such an overwhelming dilemma; I do not know where to begin."

I'm glad you asked. God has provided an answer to the problems of obesity and worldwide hunger: fasting. Specifically, let's look at the impact American church members could have if we stopped eating out so often. I discussed previously how much the restaurant business contributes to our lack of health. The caloric intake alone should deter us from going to fast-food restaurants more than once or twice a month.

However, the greatest reason to avoid eating out may be the money we would save by preparing our own healthy meals at home. The National Restaurant Association estimates that Americans spend nearly half of their family food budgets at restaurants. In 2009, that totaled almost $566 billion.[5] That is more than half a trillion dollars. What if we ate out half as much? What could groups like World Vision or Compassion International do with an extra $250 billion? They might not eradicate world hunger, but with those extra resources, surely they could save millions of lives.

Let's make this a little more personal. In 2009, the U.S. Department of Labor estimated that the average household spent $6,133 on food. Nearly half (44 percent) of that figure (or $2,668) was spent on food consumed away from home.[6] What if you cut your "eating out" budget in half? In addition, what if you fasted one day a week? That would reduce your overall food budget by 14 percent. We're talking nearly $900 a year for the average family. What if you took the money you saved and gave it to people who are dying *for* food instead of dying *from* food? World Vision claims they can feed and clothe a starving child for $30 a month. An extra $900 donation, therefore, brings sustenance to 30 children for a month. Imagine if just 11 other families would do this. You could keep those 30 kids fed all year, every year. I don't know about you, but if missing a few meals will save that many lives, I'm more than willing to do it! (And I'll be healthier to boot!)

Where to Begin

There are a number of excellent books on fasting, and I encourage you to educate yourself on this foundational Christian practice.[7] In the meantime, I'd like to give you a few tips on fasting, just to get you started.

1. Check with your family physician to ensure that you are physically able to fast.
2. Drink plenty of healthy liquids—mainly water and 100 percent fruit juices—in the days leading up to and including your fast.
3. On your first fasting day, eat a healthy breakfast, skip lunch, and eat a small dinner.
4. A week later, eat a healthy breakfast, and then skip lunch and dinner, making sure to drink lots of healthy liquids throughout the day. Each time you feel hungry, take time to pray and reflect on your walk with God.
5. Break your fast with a healthy *break-fast* the next morning. (You've just completed a 24-hour fast.)

Picking up the Keys

When I speak to teenagers, I use lots of illustrations to keep them interested in my topic. One night, while talking to our youth group about breaking the chains of addiction, I asked a police officer to bring in a set of handcuffs and place them on the stage. Next to the handcuffs, he set the keys and a 50-dollar bill. I told the students, "Officer Jones is going to take volunteers. He is going to handcuff you like he does a prisoner. If you can get yourself out of those handcuffs, you can have this 50-dollar bill. Who will volunteer?" Dozens of hands shot into the air.

I started with a few older guys. The officer clamped on the cuffs, and I chuckled as I watched the "prisoners" grimace and shake as they tried to pull their hands out of their new shackles. One young man pulled so hard that his wrists started to bleed. Another banged his wrists on the stage until he put a crack in the wood. Student after student used similar exertion until they either gave up or I made them stop for fear they were going to physically harm themselves.

After 20 minutes, complaints rumbled through the crowd. "It can't be done," someone griped; another person said, "If it were possible, people would be breaking out of prison." I assured them the task could be accomplished. Others tried. The more frustrated they grew, the more humorous it became. Officer Jones and I were laughing so hard we struggled to breathe. Finally, a seventh-grade girl who weighed less than 90 pounds walked up and said meekly, "I think I can do it." The big football players seated in the back hooted with laughter. "No way!" one exclaimed. "Make sure you put those things on tight so her little wrists don't just slide out!"

Officer Jones secured the girl's wrists with the tightest setting. She paused for a moment, looked at her wrists, picked up the keys, unlocked the handcuffs, took the 50-dollar bill, and walked back to her seat. The room erupted with laughter as several boys complained, "That's not fair." I explained that all along I had intended for someone to pick up those keys. If any of the other students had been smart enough to use them, they would have been 50 bucks richer. It was that simple.

The keys to unlocking the chains of the poor are found in the practice of fasting. This is the fast that God wants. As we abstain from unhealthy and fattening foods, we save. We save ourselves from health conditions, save ourselves from spiritual and emotional problems, save money, save our lives, and save the lives of others. Even if no other nation in the world helped us on this issue, the United States alone could effectively end world hunger by eating less, eating better and giving more. It *is* that simple.

The stage is set. God has given us every tool we need to advance justice on this planet. One thing we can do to get started is stop gorging ourselves on food. Our food chains are binding our children, churches, country and world. The key to the lock is sitting there on the stage. So is the prize. The world is watching to see if we are wise enough to pick up the keys.

So is the Maker of us all.

Questions for Discussion

1. Slow lines at the grocery store are one of my pet peeves. When it comes to waiting for something, what makes you impatient?

2. Have you ever tried some kind of fast for 24 or 48 hours? What results did you see?
3. Do you see fasting as something only for "super spiritual" people? How could it benefit you?
4. How many times a day would you estimate that you see advertisements for fast food or restaurants? What impact does this make on your outlook about food?
5. Have you ever known someone who practices fasting? Ask them about their experiences.
6. What are your struggles with your "flesh"? How might God use the practice of fasting to assist you in this area?
7. If each member or family in your congregation ate out one time less a week and donated the money to your church, how much could that generate? What could the church do with that money?

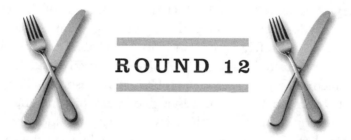

ROUND 12

It's Not Business;
It's Personal

Pawpaw's standard pre-dinner routine included sticking a needle in his stomach. Because of diabetes, my grandfather needed insulin to help him digest the government commodities lined up on his refrigerator and pantry shelves. Those brick-sized blocks of cheese affected his sugar levels. He used to mix that cheese with the powdered milk and powdered eggs Uncle Sam also provided. We ate lots of fatty foods, such as ample servings of macaroni and cheese, fried potatoes, buttermilk biscuits slathered with margarine, and pinto beans. Even though beans are a good source of protein, by the time we added lard or pork rinds for flavoring, they weren't too healthy. With many of our entrees, you could float a small boat across the grease.

I grew up in a pair of coal-driven towns in West Virginia. Various myths have sprouted over the years about my home state, particularly portrayals of us as uneducated, lazy folks who subsist on welfare. Granted, some do "game" the system and freeload their way through life, but those kinds of people exist in every state. Though neither of my grandfathers was the most erudite of men, both were incredible providers for their families in the toughest of times. Both were hard-working coal miners, but at times they earned so little that without government commodities, their families would have gone hungry during part of each month.

If low wages weren't bad enough, up until a few years before I was born, a semblance of the company store still existed. After deducting rent for their ramshackle housing (which was owned by the company), companies paid miners with "scrip." Worthless in the outside world, these coins could only be redeemed for slightly higher-priced groceries and other goods at a store owned by the same company that mined the coal. Even if you found a better deal someplace else, you couldn't take advantage of it. It was often said that once a man went down into the mines, he never came out. Given the way many of the coal companies treated their workers, that saying was true in more ways than one.

Two months after I came along, my father found a job in the mines, too. Mom was enrolled in college with hopes of becoming a teacher. The downside to their efforts was that I didn't see much of them in my formative years. Early each morning, my mother would drive me to my grandparents' house; a few hours before dark, she would come back to get me. Don't misunderstand me. I never lacked a family that provided lots of love, but we sure didn't have an abundance to eat.

While many love to romanticize tough times, I am delighted that those days are in my past. Our $50-a-month apartment left much to be desired. I can remember sticking cardboard in the holes in the walls to block the bitter winter winds howling through eastern Kanawha County. Mom and Dad have a recording of the time they asked me what I wanted for Christmas, and at age four, I replied, "All I want is a pair of shoes that don't have holes in them so my feet don't get so cold."

Because I know what it is like to be poor, I know a raw deal when I see one. Without question, the government's commodity system in the early 1970s was beyond ridiculous. I literally shudder when I think of the quality of food my grandparents received when they were out of work. These staples were so full of fat and sodium that it is a wonder any of our people lived beyond 60.

It's All About to Change

My early years' experience with government-subsidized food is one factor that has shaped my outlook on helping the poor. The other fuel for my passion has roots in an event that has no finite, human explanation. For you to fully grasp what happened, I need to share a bit about my past. My mother and father were the typical high school couple. Mom was a cheerleader and a good student. All Dad cared about was sports, getting drunk and getting in fights. More than once, police brought him home after he had been out all night.

During her senior year of high school, Mom got pregnant. Because of her slender frame and only gaining 11 pounds, she successfully hid her situation from friends and classmates. (There was much more of a stigma attached to unwed pregnancy back then.) As soon as Dad learned that she was pregnant, he took off for Columbus, Ohio. He wasn't sure what to do, but he knew he wasn't ready to get married—and he sure didn't need the responsibilities of fatherhood. Had this been a more modern era, and abortion seen as a reasonable solution to a nagging problem, who knows if I would even be alive? (Mom says she never would have chosen that option, but I'm glad we didn't have the chance to find out.)

Three days before I was born in August 1969, and for one of the few times in his young adult life, Dad decided to do the right thing. He returned from Columbus and pledged to marry Mom, although this belated decision meant their wedding didn't take place until three months after my birth. In the meantime, when Mom came home from the hospital, it was the first anyone on Dad's side of the family knew about her condition. My parents later told me that my paternal grandfather came home from work one day just as one of my aunts showed up at the house. Dad said, "Why don't y'all come in the back room? I want you to meet somebody." When my aunt asked, "Whose baby is that?" Dad replied, "It's mine."

That October, William "Bolts" Willis went to work in the mines. A month later, my parents eloped to Virginia for some quick nuptials and a one-day honeymoon. However, gainful employment and marriage didn't convert Dad to responsible fatherhood. He still drank, smoked pot, and did some other things on the side to supplement his income and provide more money for beer. My parents' was not a happy marriage.

Dad carried on his habits when our family moved to Handley, West Virginia, a little railroad town that consisted of several hundred people. Its primary reason for existence was its roundhouse, a huge train yard where rail cars owned by various companies converged before getting re-routed to their ultimate destinations—a type of Grand Central Station in the coalfields. Everyone who lived in Handley worked either for the railroads or in the coal mines. In reality, everyone lived off coal, because that was about all the trains hauled.

My parents' move to Handley proved to be providential. Our new next-door neighbors were a World War II veteran and his wife with the colorful names of Mokus and Maude. They treated us like their own family and built a foundational relationship with us that would change our lives. As they welcomed us and cared for our family, Mom and Dad had no idea just how much we would need them in the months to come.

A Crippling Disease

A few months before my fifth birthday, I began to have some severe pain in my left hip. At first my parents thought I was being overly dramatic, but after a couple of weeks, they decided to take me to a pediatrician. He ran a number of tests and took some X-rays, but could only speculate about my condition. My mother recalls, "He brought me back to his office and had a solemn look on his face. He said he wasn't sure what the problem was, but it very well could be bone cancer."

No mother ever wants to hear those words. Immediately, feelings of guilt shot like lightning through my mother's thoughts. Was God punishing her for having sex outside marriage? If so, why would God punish an innocent child? How would my father react to such horrible news? Just when it seemed like life couldn't get much worse, now she had hit rock bottom. Dad's reaction? He felt sorry for me, but told Mom, "If those are the cards you are dealt, those are the cards you are dealt. Deal with it."

Eventually an orthopedic surgeon, Dr. Bangani, diagnosed me with a rare ailment that doctors forecast would only get worse. At that time, little was known about Legg-Calve-Perthes disease, a deterioration of the hip bone caused by a lack of normal blood flow. To this day, there is no cure for the disease, and no one has identified a cause; however, some speculate that it stems from an artery in the hip closing prematurely.

By the time Dr. Bangani diagnosed the problem, I had reached stage four (today it is classified as lateral pillar class C) of the disease, which means more than 50 percent of the head of my hip socket had deteriorated.[1] Almost 40 years later, I tracked down Dr. Bangani and asked him what stage five would look like. "There is no stage five," he replied. "Once the deterioration gets to that point, it really doesn't matter. There was no medical treatment for the disease other than protecting you from harming yourself."

Following my diagnosis, I had to use a leg brace to keep the weight off my leg, because there wasn't enough of a hip socket there to keep my femur from ramming up into my pelvic area. Those were not happy days in the Willis household. Dad's heart started softening as he saw me sitting in our living room, watching all the other kids play outside. At times I would cry because of the pain; at other times I cried out of fear. I had no idea if I would ever walk again.

Rise Up and Walk

Since I had absolutely nothing to do that summer, our neighbor Maude invited me to something called Vacation Bible School (usually known by its initials, VBS). It met at the Baptist church that served as a leading gathering place in the small community of Handley. My family wasn't the church-going type, but what else was I going to do? Mom said I could go. The first time I did, the teacher spoke about Jesus healing a man who had been lame for 38 years (you can read the story in John 5:1-9). I thought, *If Jesus could heal a man who had been crippled for 38 years, then He can do the same for me*. When I went back to my parents' house, I declared, "I think Jesus is going to heal me."

Dad wasn't buying it. He wasn't too kind when the pastor came by to see him, either. The pastor had responded to my request that he visit my father "because all Daddy does is drink beer." When the pastor arrived, Dad welcomed him in and offered him a beer of his own. The pastor politely refused. My father told him he didn't care for "religious talk" and quickly cut off the conversation: "If I want to come to church, I'll come on my own. Don't waste your time up here anymore."

Over the next few months, something about my parents changed. They were overwhelmed by the love they saw from the people in that church. The town rallied around my family in our time of need. Soon, Mom began attending church every week. *If my son's going to go to church, then I'm going to take him*, she thought. Every time I returned to Handley Baptist, people told me they would pray for me and that Jesus could heal me. To someone with such a gloomy prognosis for the future, their statements shone like rays of hope into a darkened mine shaft. I believed them, even as the months drifted by and I showed no signs of improvement.

Then came Saturday morning, February 8, 1975. I was nearing six years of age and can remember many of the events of that day vividly. I had fallen asleep in our living room the night before, and Mom carried me into my bedroom. After tucking me in, she left my brace and my crutches in the opposite corner of the room. I awoke early, because of a thunderstorm outside, and called for Mom. She didn't hear me. Without thinking, I got out of bed and walked across the room to get my crutches. No sooner did I grab them with my hands than I realized: *I just walked across my room! Without crutches!* (I hadn't walked on my own in nearly eight months.) At first, I ran around the room; then I dashed out into the living room to tell my parents.

"Don't walk on that leg!" Mom screamed in alarm.

"Why not?" I asked. "I'm fine. I can walk. Jesus healed me, just like I said He would!"

That morning, my parents rushed me to see Dr. Bangani. When he got my X-rays back from the lab, he called my family in to show them the results. The young physician pointed to an X-ray from two months prior that showed continued developmental problems in my hip socket. Then he gestured at the current X-ray that showed a perfect hip with no signs of deterioration. Shaking his head, the doctor said, "I've never seen anything like it. I don't know what it is."

"I do," my father said.

As soon as we got home, Dad went to the refrigerator, removed his beer, and poured the contents down the drain. Afterwards, he said, "I'm never going to drink again." The next morning, he went to church and pledged to follow the Jesus who had healed his son. My parents took me to church every Sunday morning, Sunday night and Wednesday night for the next 13 years. We even went to church while we were on vacation!

Those who have never known the joy of healing or seen their families transformed may be skeptical of such stories. I don't blame you. Even though I experienced it myself, I still wondered about the disease and the facts of my case. That's why I made the effort to contact Dr. Bangani after all those years. As we discussed the details of my childhood disease, he said, "Today, it is not that uncommon to see a child recover from Perthes, but going from stage four to walking in two months is medically impossible."

I still wanted to know more, so I called a few friends in orthopedics and discussed my abnormal recovery. "The miracle was not so much that you walked again," one said. "If the onset of Legg-Perthes occurs before the age of six, the odds of someone recovering don't delve into the world of the miraculous. But you're usually looking at three to five years until you begin to walk without the aid of crutches. It's the speed at which your body regenerated the bone that is so rare."

Whether there is another explanation for my healing, I don't know. But looking back, I would ask: Which is the greater miracle? Was it what happened to my leg or what happened in my dad's heart? Was it the resiliency of my hip socket or the metamorphosis of my family's future? Without question, the lives of both my parents were miraculously transformed. Both rose from impoverished, dysfunctional environments to positions of significant responsibility. After teaching high school and college English for 16 years, Mom became a curriculum specialist for Kanawha County schools, supervising teachers in language arts and developing reading strategies. Dad was eventually appointed to oversee the West Virginia Department of Energy's enforcement of mine safety regulations and also served as an advisor to the governor. Most importantly for me, both became leaders in our church. My dad was like the Pied Piper when it came to bringing neighborhood kids to church, and Mom taught Sunday School every single week.

Stepping into Normal Life

My healing marked the start of a normal life. Now I could run and play the way other kids could. Given Dad's love of athletics, I quickly warmed to the ballfields and played high school sports. My constant activity burned up lots of calories—which was a good thing, since we continued eating plenty of commodity cheese. When Dad started in the mines, he made just enough money to put him out of range for government assistance, but my grandparents shared their provisions with us. Almost all the families in the railroad and coal towns where I grew up shared food with each other, making poor nutrition a community-wide problem.

Naturally, given the reliance on commodities in our area, our school had a good share of overweight kids, although in the early to mid-1980s that wasn't as big an issue as it is now. I never knew exactly how many were living on government assistance, but personal observation told me that most of my schoolmates were. Thanks to Mom's and Dad's frequent promotions, we had escaped their ranks by the time I got to high school, but I still empathized with everyone else. Back then, the school handed out wood chips to everyone who received free or partially subsidized meals. I noticed when kids came through the line that they would deposit the chips—which they received that morning during home room—in a basket. By the end of the lunch period, the basket would be stuffed full.

At least 80 percent of my classmates used those wood markers. For them, those meals represented a lifeline. Friends who got to school late because they forgot to set their alarm clocks would tell me how much they hated to miss breakfast, because that was the only breakfast they ever had. Even those who made it on time sometimes confided in me that they didn't have much food at home. I knew they didn't own much, because they wore the same outfit every other day, alternating between their only two sets of school clothes.

These poor kids weren't an abstraction—someone I might have just heard about who was down on his or her luck. My senior year of high school, I asked the leading scorer on our basketball team what he was doing for Christmas. "We can't afford Christmas dinner," he replied. I went home and told my parents, who helped me gather up a turkey, dressing, mashed potatoes and green beans for his family. When I got to their apartment, I took the food into the kitchen. I opened the refrigerator, and all I found was a partially filled jug of water. *Man, this isn't right*, I thought. *How can we have people living like this in the United States of America?*

Because of that early-life experience, my heart aches for children in similar circumstances. Although I have since earned my Ph.D., and my family lives in a comfortable, three-bedroom home in one of the nicer areas of town, when our church sponsors programs at the local elementary school, I recognize kids who come from modest backgrounds because of the clothes they wear or the shyness they display. Then there are the obese youngsters whose weight makes them automatic targets for ridicule. While not all of these children necessarily come from poor homes, I always wonder how many rely on the same kind of commodities that I used to eat.

Here We Go Again

There is another reason I identify with kids from poor homes. After four years at West Virginia University, four years of graduate studies at one of the nation's leading seminaries, and graduating with honors from that seminary, I never dreamed of needing government help again. Oh, I had my chance to sample comfortable suburban life. One wealthy church in Richardson, Texas—just outside Dallas—offered me more than $60,000 a year to become its youth pastor. While I was mulling over that offer, a church in southern West Virginia called. The head of their search committee said they had been looking for a youth pastor for three years, but hadn't been able to persuade anyone to come.

When Dee and I drove back to visit the church, God tugged at my heartstrings. The congregation's members were the same kind of folks I grew up with. Indeed, a few of them were part of my extended family. I wanted to help these kids, who were just like I had been. Many never had a youth pastor to help guide them through adolescence. Few had been 30 miles outside of their hometown. They had never taken mission trips to places like Chicago or Washington, DC, where they could share the love of Christ while learning that others face challenges, too. After our visit, I told my wife, "I think this is where God wants us."

To her credit, Dee agreed. That was a major step. Unlike me, she came from a more affluent family—her father's salary had enabled her mom to stay at home full-time. Her father was a corporate pilot, and most of her friends' parents were businessmen, doctors or lawyers. (She had never even heard of commodity cheese until she met me.) To put me through seminary, Dee worked as a teacher in an inner-city school. I promised that if she supported me through seminary, I would never ask her to work outside the home again. When she agreed to the deal, she never dreamed it would involve moving back to West Virginia in her sixth month of pregnancy, while I went to work for the princely sum of $20,000 a year and no medical benefits.

It wasn't long before I started wondering how we were going to pay our bills and raise our first son, Titus, on such a meager income. Since we were living much like the people in our church, one day I commented to a member, "You know, we don't know how to make it on my salary and try to raise a child, too."

"You can get on WIC," she replied.

WIC stands for the Women, Infants and Children's program that provides food vouchers for low-income families. I didn't know much about it, other than that it was just a step above food stamps.

"Well, I don't know if we'll qualify for that," I said. However, I was ready to try anything. Titus had to eat! To my surprise, we qualified by a wide margin—I could have made $10,000 more a year and still received government assistance. After we passed the review process, I went to the store with Dee to keep an eye on our son while she shopped for groceries. An aerobics instructor in college, my fitness-oriented wife wanted to buy healthy food for our baby, who had passed the breast-feeding stage. To her dismay, she learned that WIC vouchers could be used for things like eggs, milk, peanut butter, sugar-laden fruit drinks and cereal. Lots of cereal—we could buy three or four boxes a week. However, the list included no fresh fruits and very few vegetables.

Here we are, getting government assistance, but the food the government is giving us isn't what we need for our baby, I thought. *Why in the world can we buy corn meal and all kinds of cereal, but we can't go over to the produce section and buy a banana or an apple? Something is wrong with this picture.* Holding our son as I stood in the grocery store aisle, I realized this was exactly what my parents had experienced. All they could afford to feed me were the standard, carb-loaded staples. It felt like stepping into a time warp.

Don't get me wrong. I was thankful for the help we received during that challenging time in our lives. Looking back, I realize there was no way we could have served at that church without government assistance.

Besides, living that life as an adult—if only for a short while—reminded me what it was like to grow up on the other side of the tracks. There is a world that consists of the working poor, and I have lived there twice.

This is why I take the push for healthy food so seriously. I was one of those kids eating processed foods with government help. Our three children received food through WIC. I know what it is like to want to feed your children decent food and not be able to afford it. But today, standing where I stand now, I wonder why our government has the ability to provide our children with healthy foods, but instead gives them starches, fat, salt and mystery meat. Instead of helping our children avoid health problems, we are pushing them in that direction.

The Need for Reform

Fortunately, signs of reform are in the air. The WIC program was implemented nationally in 1974. In 2009, New York became the first state to implement major changes to its program, adding such items as whole grains, low-fat milk, fruits, vegetables, tofu and brown rice to its list of approved foods. Other states followed in 2010. Ironically, as WIC steps toward a healthier future, a comment from the director of a community health center shows the battle we still face to overcome the waves of subsidized corn products and fast-food advertising. "Originally, the food package was meant to eliminate vitamin deficiencies," said Pam Harbin of the Ryan Community Health Center in New York. "But now it is no longer a vitamin deficiency problem. It's over-nutrition that we have to deal with."[2]

With powerful forces backing the status quo, educating mothers and the rest of society about the benefits of healthy eating will be an ongoing challenge. So will efforts to reform government policies so that we can tip the scales toward fruits and vegetables. People who scream about government interference in free markets usually don't recognize that Uncle Sam is already interfering. It is just a question of whose side he takes. As so often happens with political policy, those who scream the loudest or can afford the best lobbyists come out on top.

As I see it, current policy allocates tax dollars to producing crops that wind up in processed foods. Then our taxes purchase those foods on the back end through programs like WIC and food stamps. We pay a third time for the processed food-like substances through the school lunch program. That is followed 30 to 40 years later by a fourth set of bills when the people who ate all that processed food develop heart disease and other medical problems. Some of them are on Medicaid as adults, and when they reach 65, government-subsidized Medicare steps in to complete the cycle. Is it any wonder we grapple with trillion-dollar deficits?

My mother, Margie Willis, represents the end result of the poor nutrition and ill-advised medical care that have long typified small coal towns. Struck by strange symptoms of tiredness and constant fatigue in her mid-forties, she struggled through half of one more school year before taking a medical leave that stretched into permanent disability. Starting with rheumatic fever at the age of three, her long list of ailments can't be traced to a single factor.

However, she believes a lack of proper nutrition played a major role. Growing up, she ate a steady diet of pinto beans and fried potatoes, with the occasional Sunday dinner adding chicken and mashed potatoes. While the family garden provided some vegetables during the summer, no green foods ever appeared on her plate during long winters. "Sometimes I ate coal ashes because I was so hungry," she laments. "Looking back, I'm embarrassed by it, but what else was I to do? My biggest regret is that, once my husband and I climbed out of poverty, we did like most Americans and ate fast food four to five times a week. There was no excuse for it. My priorities were in the wrong place. Now I'm paying the price."

There is no telling exactly what difference good nutrition would have made in my mom's health, but I believe its absence lies at the heart of many of her problems—like the irritable bowel syndrome she developed in college and allergies diagnosed after she turned 22. The latter caused severe headaches that would send her to bed for a week or two at a time. It took visits to several doctors to discover that she was allergic to wheat, gluten, bread, milk, eggs and anything in the kale family, as well as mold, pet hair and tree dander. Later, she needed treatment for a nerve disorder. She also came down with Lyme disease in 2004 after getting bitten by a deer tick. While she can't prove it, Mom believes a weakened immune system made her susceptible to the disease.

Today, she looks back on her nutritional choices with regret. "I didn't take care of myself until I got sick in my mid-forties," Mom reflects. "Now I know what it takes to live a healthy life, but the damage has been done." Failing a healing miracle of her own, my mother's chances for a normal life are slim. Though she's only 49 years older than my youngest son, I've never seen her pick him up and hold him.

Go and Make Disciples

While my mother's situation looks bleak, I still hold out hope for the children of our world. But at times, I feel like America is doing everything it can to perpetuate our consumerism on the world's developing nations. In early 2011, I visited the Copperbelt region of Zambia with the hopes of partnering with an orphanage there and perhaps even adopting a child of our own. As I was working on the purchase of some land, I noticed some cornfields nearby. I have no idea why, but I asked the local missionary how farmers in the area grow their corn.

"There was a day when the Zambians grew their own corn and kept enough seed to plant the following year," said Sandra Hayashida, an instructor at Zambian International Theological College. "But now they use American corn that has been modified so the seed from the harvest is only good for eating. If they try to use the offspring of the original seed, it gives such a lower yield, it's not worth the time and effort to plant it."

Intrigued, I later spoke with a Zambian farmer, who explained to me that Zambian agriculture was doing fine just a few decades ago, but then some companies from the United States came in to "aid" them with a genetically altered seed that yields about 20 percent more than what they were using. There was only one catch: The seed was useless if they wanted to store some for future planting. They would have to use the corn from America every year thereafter.

This seed, which had been subsidized by American tax dollars, was so inexpensive that Zambian farmers jumped at the chance to make a quick buck. Those who used to grow other vegetables also boarded the corn bandwagon and only planted the genetically altered corn. When harvest time came around, so much corn came to market that it drove the cost down to where farmers with smaller crops did not make enough profit to make ends meet. (Sound familiar?) In order to survive, the farmers who still had unaltered Zambian corn had to sell or eat the seed they were saving for next year.

So let's say you are a farmer in Zambia, and because cheap American corn has flooded your market, instead of making four dollars a bushel, this year you make two dollars a bushel. You were already living hand-to-mouth, so after a couple of seasons like this, in order to get your family through the winter, you have to sell your land to the farmers who use American corn. (Unlike in America, the Zambian government doesn't have the money to bail you out!) Pretty soon, you and most of your friends are out of business, but at least you can work another job and buy corn for two dollars a bushel. That's a cheap way to feed your family.

But wait! You show up at the market, and now that all the competition is gone, the genetically altered American corn has been raised to $3.50 a bushel. You can buy some, and it will be good for one harvest, but come next year you'll be back with your hat in your hand. To make matters worse, you will have to lease back the land you sold to the other farmers, just so you have a place to plant your new-bought corn. Sounds like the days of the company store and scrip, doesn't it?

I wish this were a fictional story, but it is not. Today, the unemployment rate in Zambia is nearly 80 percent, and people struggle to survive. At most meals, children receive a few ounces of nshima, a cheap version of what we would call corn meal. They eat nshima for breakfast, lunch and dinner. It would be nice to have some other vegetable options, but cheap American corn has run most other crop farmers out of business. So while people are able to survive on corn meal, their oily and starch-filled diet has also led to a nutritionally deficient population that struggles with heart disease and diabetes.

At the heart of all this misery stands young Penelope. This eight-year-old girl represents a nation of orphans, most of whom have lost their parents to the AIDS virus. Years ago, due to the plummeting agricultural markets, many women resorted to selling their bodies just to get their children something to eat. Soon young girls were doing the same. The result, in 2011, is a country where nearly a third of the population aged 18 to 35 has AIDS, and close to 20 percent of the children don't have a living parent. Penelope is one of more than a million children who are just like her.[3] For most countries in Africa, the story is the same.

While most of Africa's problems are not the fault of Americans, that doesn't excuse the fact that some American companies have become rich and powerful by exploiting the African people. The practice of underselling corn makes me think of the passage in Jeremiah 5:27-29, where the prophet proclaims, " 'Like cages full of birds, their houses are full of deceit; they have become rich and powerful and have grown fat and sleek. Their evil deeds have no limit; they do not plead the case of the fatherless to win it; they do not defend the rights of the poor. Should I not punish them for this?' declares the LORD. 'Should I not avenge myself on such a nation as this?' "

Are those harsh words? Absolutely! And whether or not we individually bear responsibility for Africa's plight, as a nation we have—at best—

turned a blind eye to the businesses that have grown fat by failing to promote the cause of the fatherless and defend the cause of the poor. If we continue with this behavior, we have God's promise that He will act. He will not sit idly by and continue to watch us exploit the poor so we can fatten up our children. Something has to change!

So please understand, when I talk about the importance of improving nutrition in this world, it's not business; it's personal. This book isn't about business either—I'm having the proceeds donated to our church to support various ministries, including the one in Zambia, and, Lord willing, Dee and I may find a way to adopt young Penelope. For me, this is *very* personal. It's about my grandparents, my mother, my wife, my children, my congregation, my former schoolmates and my Zambian friends. Most importantly, it is about my God. I know Jesus sheds a tear as our gluttonous food habits kill our own children while starving others who have nothing at all. Sometimes it makes me sad. Sometimes it makes me angry. But it always makes me want to fight.

A Word from Rocky Balboa

Like most every other American boy of the 1970s and '80s, I grew up watching the *Rocky* movies. When I was in fifth grade, our entire class went wild in the theater when Rocky Balboa battled round after round to defeat Apollo Creed and capture the heavyweight championship of the world. Up until 2006, *Rocky II* was my favorite of all. However, in his last installment, Sylvester Stallone came up with one of his best scripts (I know, I know, no Academy Awards, but hey, it's Rocky). In *Rocky Balboa*, the old boxer was well past the end of his career, and he was trying to muster up the strength for one more fight. His son, who was failing at his own business endeavors, encouraged his dad to give up the idea of fighting. After all, Rocky was old, and the path to victory was too steep for him to climb.

That was when Rocky gave his greatest speech of all (cue Rocky music here), in which he proclaimed that the world wasn't all sunshine and rainbows, but a mean, nasty place that would beat you to your knees and keep you there if you let it. While nobody would hit as hard as life, he reminded his son that it wasn't how hard he hit that mattered, but how hard he could get hit and keep moving forward. That's how winning was done, proclaimed the great fighter who never knew the word quit. "Now, if you know what you're worth, then go out and get what you're worth," Rocky exhorted. "But you gotta be willing to take the hit, and not pointing fingers saying you ain't where you are because of him, or her, or anybody. Cowards do that and that ain't you. You're better than that!"[4]

Rocky is right! We are better than this! America is better than this. Our schools are better than this. Your community is better than this. Your church is better than this. Your family is better than this. YOU are better than this!

This fight is not about how hard we will hit, but how hard we can get hit—and keep moving forward. Whatever you do, don't quit! With God's favor, this food fight is a battle that will be won.

Questions for Discussion

1. Can you relate to my experience of growing up eating commodity cheese and pork-laced pinto beans? How is poor nutrition linked to poverty? How do government programs contribute to the problem of obesity?

2. Does it concern you that the federal government helps subsidize crops that often contribute to health problems, but does not adequately subsidize fruits and vegetables? What do you see as a possible solution?

3. My family might never have changed if it weren't for my crippling childhood disease. Why does it often take something tragic to change our direction in life? How might this concept relate to your dietary choices?

4. Do you know anyone who can be classified as "working poor" (or do you fall into this category yourself)? What kind of diet do they (or you) follow? What kinds of medical problems do they (or you) have?

5. Clearly, governmental subsidies are putting our health at risk here at home. How does our international trade also contribute to world hunger? Do you think God is concerned about our treatment of developing nations? What can we do about it?

6. As you have read this book, what specific and measurable plans have you established? What is your timeline for accomplishing your plans? Who will help keep you accountable to achieving these goals?

7. Whenever we are challenged with new knowledge, we are responsible to pass that information on to others who need it as well. Name some close friends who should read this book. How can you get this information in their hands?

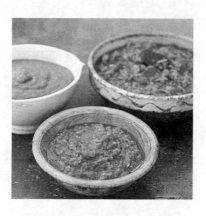

RECIPES
BY JAMIE OLIVER

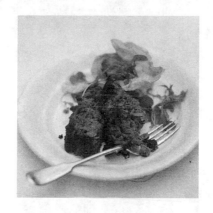

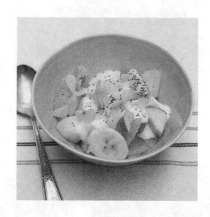

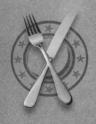

"FULL OF VEG" TOMATO BASE SAUCE

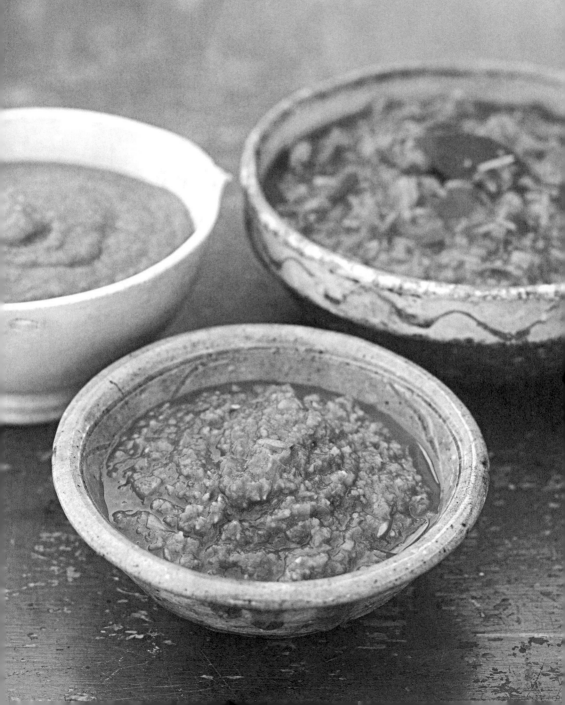

"Full of Veg" Tomato Base Sauce

This is a great sauce to have up your sleeve. It will have a lovely, sweet flavor, just like tomatoes. I've whizzed the sauce up with a stick blender to disguise the vegetables for kids, but after they get used to eating it, you can whiz them up a bit less each time until, eventually, you won't have to whiz it at all. This recipe makes quite a big batch. I tend to make loads at one time, let it cool completely, then bag it up and freeze it. Serves 6 to 8, with plenty of leftovers.

- **2 small onions**
- **1 small leek**
- **2 stalks of celery**
- **2 red bell peppers**
- **2 zucchini**
- **2 carrots**
- **olive oil**
- **large pinch of dried oregano**
- **2 bay leaves**
- **1 small butternut squash**
- **4 x 14½-oz. tins plum tomatoes**
- **sea salt**
- **freshly ground black pepper**

Peel and chop the onions. Trim and wash the leek and celery, making sure you wash the leek well. Deseed and chop the bell peppers, then coarsely grate the zucchinis and carrots.

Heat a large saucepan (big enough to hold all the ingredients) over a medium heat. Add a good splash of olive oil then add all the chopped veg along with the oregano and bay leaves. Cook the whole lot slowly for about 20 minutes with the lid on, or until all the vegetables are nice and soft but without any color at all.

Meanwhile, carefully peel the butternut squash then cut it in half and remove the seeds. Coarsely grate it. Add the tinned tomatoes, grated squash, 2 cups of water and a pinch of salt and pepper to the vegetables. Bring to boil and simmer gently for about 30 minutes, or until the squash is soft.

Fish out the bay leaves and allow the sauce to cool slightly before blitzing with a stick blender until nice and smooth. Have a taste and season with a little more salt and pepper if needed.

Recipe © Jamie Oliver, photography © David Loftus.

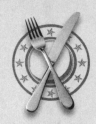

MEATLOAF

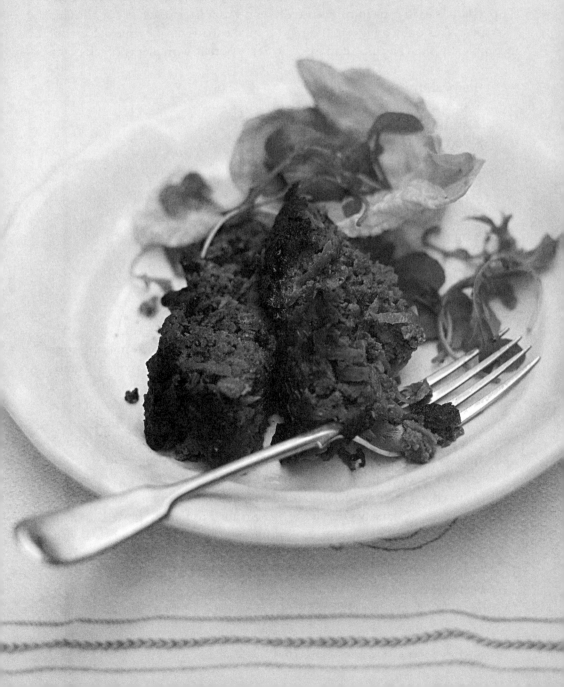

Meatloaf

Meatloaf is a great family favorite and it's really easy and cheap to make. It's a good meal to make in advance and has loads of flavor. It doesn't have to be made with beef or turkey, try it with lamb, chicken or even pork for a twist on the old classic. Serves 4.

1 tbsp. olive oil, plus extra for greasing the pan
1 red onion, peeled and finely chopped
1 large carrot, grated
¼ cup breadcrumbs
1 large free-range egg
⅛ cup (1 x 5-oz. can) tomato paste
2 tbsp. Dijon mustard
½ tsp. dried thyme
1 tsp. Worcestershire sauce
1 lb. lean ground turkey or beef

Preheat the oven to 375°F. Lightly grease a baking sheet and set it aside. Heat a sauté pan over medium heat and pour in a lug [tablespoon] of oil. Add the onion and cook for 5 to 10 minutes, or until soft. Stir in the carrot and tip into a bowl to cool.

When the veggies are cool, add the breadcrumbs, eggs, tomato paste, mustard, thyme and Worcestershire sauce. With clean hands, give everything a good mix, then add the ground turkey or beef. Scrunch and mix everything together really well. Tip the mixture out onto the baking sheet, then pat and mould it into a long oval shape.

Bake for 40 minutes. To tell if the meatloaf is done, poke the thickest part with a knife—the juices that trickle out should be clear, not pink. Serve hot. I like to serve it with a little bit of sour cream or plain yogurt and a nice crunchy salad, and to make a bigger meal of it you can add some guacamole, fluffy rice or tortillas. Or, you could try serving it with home-made tomato sauce spooned over the top for a bit of a change.

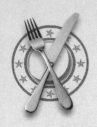

SIMPLEST FRUIT SALAD

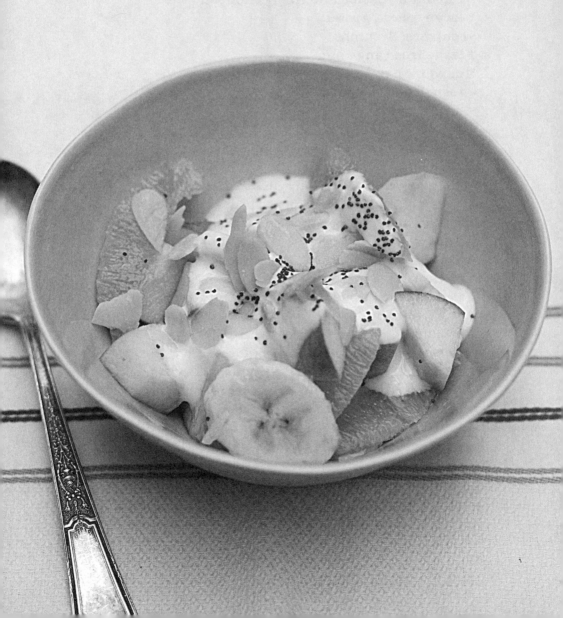

Simplest Fruit Salad

This is a very simple and delicious recipe. Start with the freshest fruit you can find and you'll wonder why you don't make this everyday! Fruit salad is the best way to celebrate seasonal fruit so feel free to vary what I've used here depending on the time of year—buying fruit that's in season will ensure you have the best flavors possible. Serves 4.

1 cup plain yogurt
2 tbsp. honey
2 oranges
2 bananas
1 apple
1 tsp. poppy seeds
4 tbsp. sliced almonds, or your favorite nuts

Stir the yogurt and honey together in a small bowl.

Top and tail the oranges. Stand them up on a cutting board and cut off the peel and the white pith right down to the orange. Work over a bowl to catch the juices and cut the orange segments free, letting them drop right into the bowl. Squeeze the juice from what's left of the oranges into the bowl.

Wash the apple, cut it into quarters and cut out the core and seeds. Cut the apples into chunks and add them to the bowl. Peel and slice the bananas and toss them with the other fruit. Spoon the fruit into four bowls and spoon some of the yogurt over each. Sprinkle the poppy seeds and almonds over the yogurt.

Recipe © Jamie Oliver, photography © Dan Jones

Resources

I appreciate Regal Books/Gospel Light for being one of the leading Christian publishers addressing the Church's total health. I strongly encourage readers to visit their website (www.gospellight.com) and check out their "Healthy Living" resources, which integrate faith and fitness. Outside of the trusted publications from Regal, if you want to further educate yourself about the food you are eating and its effect on your health, here are my top 10 recommendations. Each will arm you with the knowledge you need to win your food fight.

Recommended Reading List

Books

1. *A Hunger for God: Desiring God Through Fasting and Prayer* by John Piper. The well-known pastor and teacher describes how fasting can help us in our pursuit of God, leaving us deeply satisfied. I like most of Piper's books, but this work is a must-read for all people of faith.

2. *What to Eat* by Marion Nestle. The guru of healthy food, this New York University professor takes a trip through the grocery store, showing how advertising and other methods encourage us to eat more than we need and cause a detrimental impact to our health. This reference book is foundational for understanding the terminology of our food system.

3. *The Family Dinner: Great Ways to Connect with Your Kids, One Meal at a Time* by Laurie David. A film and TV producer, David writes about how family dinners can help parents address modern-day challenges of raising children in a technological age. If America's food fight is going to be won, it will find victory around the family dinner table.

4. *The Omnivore's Dilemma: A Natural History of Four Meals* by Michael Pollan. A long-time writer for the *New York Times* and a journalism instructor, Pollan traces meals from four distinct sources to show how the modern food chain is damaging to our health.

5. *The End of Overeating: Taking Control of the Insatiable American Appetite* by David Kessler. Kessler, a former Food and Drug Administration commissioner, discusses how food companies push infinite combinations of salt, fat and sugar to stimulate our desire to overeat. The information in the first 100 pages changed the way my family eats out.

6. *Food Politics: How the Food Industry Influences Nutrition and Health* by Marion Nestle. Nestle, a nutrition professor, details how the food industry influences our dietary choices to the detriment of our health.

7. *Food Rules: An Eater's Manual* by Michael Pollan. The author provides a handbook with straightforward guidelines about eating wisely, reminding readers that eating doesn't have to be complicated.

8. *Fasting for Spiritual Breakthrough* by Elmer Towns. This long-time Bible professor spells out the benefits that come from fasting and explains how this discipline can help people draw closer to God.

9. *Made to Crave* by Lysa Terkeurst. This book, written from a deeply spiritual perspective, has helped a number of women in our church overcome their insatiable appetite for food and replace that craving with a deeper hunger for God.

10. *In Defense of Food: An Eater's Manifesto* by Michael Pollan. Leave the processed food on the shelf and follow Pollan's recommendations for fresh, healthy eating. It's hard to go wrong with food the way God created it.

Documentaries

Food Inc. If you don't want to read Pollan's *Omnivore's Dilemma,* at least take the time to watch this documentary. Filmmaker Robert Kenner lifts the lid on America's food industry, showing how this highly mechanized machine often puts profits ahead of our health, the farmers, workers and our environment.

Forks Over Knives. This film follows the journeys of two researchers who uncovered how a plant-based diet of whole foods can help prevent and reverse such degenerative diseases as heart disease, Type 2 diabetes, and several kinds of cancer.

Websites

Winningthefoodfight.com and *fbckenova.com*. This is my website on which I share updated stories of the continuing food fight in the Tri-state area. My sermons on obesity, integrating faith and justice and many other topics can be found here.

JamieOliver.com. Jamie is at the forefront of the food battle. Links to hundreds of recipes and other food-related issues can be found here. Go to the "Food Revolution" link to find hundreds of resources.

Slowfood.com. Again, hundreds of resources right at your fingertips.

Endnotes

Round 1: The Call

1. Greta Kilmer, MS, Henry Roberts, PhD, Elizabeth Hughes, DrPH, et al, "Surveillance of Certain Health Behaviors and Conditions Among States and Selected Local Areas—Behavioral Risk Factor Surveillance System (BRFSS), United States, 2006," Centers for Disease Control, 15 August 2008, http://www.cdc.gov/mmwr/preview/mmwrhtml/ss5707a1.htm.
2. "Obesity Bigger Threat Than Terrorism?" CBS News, 1 March 2006, http://www.cbsnews.com/stories/2006/03/01/health/main1361849.shtml.
3. "A Surgeon General's Opinion: Obesity Is America's #1 Health Concern," Revolution Health, 25 April 2008, http://www.revolutionhealth.com/blogs/valjonesmd/posts_by_category/weight-disorders/obesity.
4. Morgan Spurlock, *Don't Eat This Book: Fast Food and the Supersizing of America* (New York: Berkley Books, 2006), p. 14.
5. John Robbins, *The Food Revolution: How Your Diet Can Help Save Your Life and Our World* (San Francisco: Conari Press, 2011), p. 38.
6. Spurlock, *Don't Eat This Book*, p. 15.
7. David A. Kessler, M.D., *The End of Overeating: Taking Control of the Insatiable American Appetite* (Emmaus, PA: Rodale Books, 2009), p. 94.
8. "National Health Expenditure Projections 2010-2020," Centers for Medicare & Medicaid Services, https://www.cms.gov/nationalhealthexpenddata/downloads/proj2010.pdf.
9. Linda Bloom, "Study shows high obesity rate for clergy," *United Methodist News Service*, 1 June 2010, http://www.umc.org/site/apps/nlnet/content3.aspx?c=lwL4KnN1LtH&b=2789393&ct=8419943, accessed September 2011.
10. Eryn Sun, "Firm Faith, Fat Body? Study Finds High Rate of Obesity among Religious," *Christian Post*, 24 March 2011, http://www.christianpost.com/news/firm-faith-fat-body-study-finds-high-rate-of-obesity-among-religious-49568/print.html, accessed September 2011.
11. R.C. Whitaker, J.A. Wright, M.S. Pepe, K.D. Seidel and W.H. Deitz, "Predicting Obesity in Young Adulthood from Childhood and Parental Obesity," *New England Journal of Medicine* 1997, 37(13): 869-873.

Round 3: Does God Really Care?

1. Although we are not bound by the Mosaic Law today, the overwhelming number of dietary laws in the Hebrew Bible demonstrates how important proper nutrition was for the people of Israel.

Round 5: The Man in the Mirror

1. David A. Kessler, M.D., *The End of Overeating: Taking Control of the Insatiable American Appetite* (Emmaus, PA: Rodale Books, 2009), p. 14.
2. Ibid., p. 11.
3. Ibid., p. 31.
4. Ibid., p. 94.

Round 6: There's No Place Like Home

1. David A. Kessler, M.D., *The End of Overeating: Taking Control of the Insatiable American Appetite* (Emmaus, PA: Rodale Books, 2009), p. 83.
2. Michael Pollan, *The Omnivore's Dilemma* (New York: Penguin Press, 2006), p. 3.
3. This information comes from the McDonald's website. See http://nutrition.mcdonalds.com/nutritionexchange/nutritionfacts.pdf.
4. "Chain Restaurants Charged With Promoting 'X-treme Eating,' " Center for Science in the Public Interest, 26 February 2007, www.cspinet.org/new/200702233.html.
5. "Research on the benefits of family meals," Dakota County Department of Public Health, updated 08 April 2011, http://www.co.dakota.mn.us/Departments/PublicHealth/Projects/ResearchFamilyMeals.htm.

6. Laurie David, *The Family Dinner* (New York: Grand Central Life & Style, 2010), p. 12.
7. Ibid.
8. Jeanie Lerche Davis, "Family Dinners Are Important," WebMD, July 17, 2007. http://children.web md.com/guide/family-dinners-are-important.
9. Barbara H. Fiese, Ph.D, and Marlene Schwartz, Ph.D., "Reclaiming the Family Table: Mealtimes and Child Health and Wellbeing," *Social Policy Report*, 2008, http://www.srcd.org/index.php? option=com_docman&task=doc_download&Itemid=&gid=359.
10. Dr. Harvey Harp, cited in David, *The Family Dinner*, p. 12.
11. For information about this program, visit www.coolrunning.com.

Round 8: It's Taking a Village
1. Michael Pollan, *The Omnivore's Dilemma* (New York: Penguin Press, 2006), p. 179.
2. Michael Pollan, *In Defense of Food: An Eater's Manifesto* (New York: Penguin Non-Classics, 2009), p. 1.

Round 9: Back to School
1. Marion Nestle, *Food Politics* (Berkeley, CA: University of California Press, 2002), p. 188.
2. Ibid., p. 77.
3. Michael Pollan, *In Defense of Food: An Eater's Manifesto* (New York: Penguin Non-Classics, 2009), p. 24.
4. Nestle, *Food Politics*, p. 76.
5. "Mission statement," U.S. Department of Agriculture, http://www.usda.gov/wps/portal/usda/us dahome?navid=MISSION_STATEMENT.
6. "What does FDA do?" U.S. Food and Drug Administration, http://www.fda.gov/AboutFDA/ Transparency/Basics/ucm194877.htm.
7. Nestle, *Food Politics*, p. 100.
8. Roni Caryn Rabin, "Childhood: Obesity and School Lunches," *The New York Times*, 4 February 2011, http://www.nytimes.com/2011/02/08/health/research/08childhood.html.
9. Jane Black, "School Lunch Is Not the Answer," The Hive, 24 February 2011, http://hive.slate.com/ hive/time-to-trim/article/school-lunch-is-not-the-answer.
10. Morgan Spurlock, *Don't Eat This Book: Fast Food and the Supersizing of America* (New York: Berkley Books, 2006), pp. 126-127.

Round 10: The Politics of Food
1. Caroline E. Mayer and Amy Joyce, "The Escalating Obesity Wars," *The Washington Post*, 27 April 2005, http://www.washingtonpost.com/wp-dyn/content/article/2005/04/26/AR2005042601259.html.
2. Marion Nestle, *Food Politics* (Berkeley, CA: University of California Press, 2002), p. 11.
3. Ibid., p. 2.
4. Morgan Spurlock, *Don't Eat This Book: Fast Food and the Supersizing of America* (New York: Berkley Books, 2006), p. 18.
5. Michael Pollan, *The Omnivore's Dilemma* (New York: Penguin Press, 2006), p. 53.
6. Spurlock, *Don't Eat This Book*, p. 19.
7. Marion Nestle, "Three reports: eat more fruits and vegetables," Food Politics, 11 November 2010, http://www.foodpolitics.com/2010/11/three-reports-eat-more-fruits-and-vegetables/.
8. Nestle, *Food Politics*, p. 22.
9. Ibid.
10. Mark Bittman, *Food Matters: A Guide to Conscious Eating with More Than 75 Recipes* (New York: Simon & Schuster, 2009), p. 26.
11. Pollan, *The Omnivore's Dilemma*, p. 82.
12. Spurlock, *Don't Eat This Book*, p. 104.
13. Ibid.
14. Bittman, *Food Matters*, p. 22.
15. Ibid., p. 1.
16. Andrew L. Dannenberg, MD, MPH, Deron C. Burton, MD, JD, MPH, and Richard J. Jackson, MD, MPH, "Economic and environmental costs of obesity," *American Journal of Preventive Medicine*, vol. 27, no. 3, October 2004, p. 264.

17. John Robbins, *The Food Revolution: How Your Diet Can Help Save Your Life and Our World* (San Francisco: Conari Press, 2011), p. 122. Irradiation was allowed for school foods starting in 2004.
18. Ibid.
19. Dr. Don Colbert, *The Seven Pillars of Health* (Lake Mary, FL: Siloam Press, 2006), p. 102.
20. Ibid.
21. Ibid.
22. Pollan, *The Omnivore's Dilemma*, p. 201.
23. See the resources section at the end of this book for suggested readings on these issues.
24. See Marion Nestle, *Food Politics,* http://www.foodpolitics.com/2010/11/three-reports-eat-more-fruits-and-vegetables/. For more ideas on government involvement, read *Food Politics* by Marion Nestle.

Round 11: Life in the Fast(ing) Lane

1. Some may argue that this statement is made within the context of combating demonic forces. I would ask, "What is more demonic than a system that simultaneously kills children with too much food and withholds sustenance from children dying of starvation?"
2. Elmer L. Towns, *The Daniel Fast for Spiritual Breakthrough* (Ventura, CA: Regal Books, 2010), p. 15.
3. Jordan S. Rubin, *The Maker's Diet* (New York: Berkley Publishing Group, 2005), p. 171.
4. "Hunger Facts," World Vision, http://www.worldvision.org/content.nsf/learn/hunger-facts, accessed September 2011.
5. "Pocket Factbook," National Restaurant Association, 2009. http://www.restaurant.org/pdfs/research/2009Factbook.pdf.
6. "How The Average U.S. Consumer Spends Their Paycheck" Visual Economics, http://www.visualeconomics.com/how-the-average-us-consumer-spends-their-paycheck/, accessed September 2011.
7. Some of my favorite readings on fasting are *Fasting for Spiritual Breakthrough* by Elmer Towns, *A Hunger for God* by John Piper, and *Fasting* by Scot McKnight. For a basic overview of fasting, check out Bill Bright's articles on Campus Crusade for Christ's website at http://www.ccci.org/training-and-growth/devotional-life/personal-guide-to-fasting/index.htm.

Round 12: It's Not Business; It's Personal

1. Ali Nawaz Khan, "Legg-Calve-Perthes Disease Imaging" Medscape Reference, http://emedicine.medscape.com/article/410482-overview.
2. Kafi Drexel, "State Revamps WIC Program With Healthier Focus" NY1.com, January 26, 2009, http:///www.ny1.com/content/ny1_living/92837/state-revamps-wic-program-with-healthier-focus/, accessed September 2011.
3. "Orphans of AIDS in our hands," Zambia Orphans of AIDS, http://www.zambiaorphans.org/Documents/ZOA-Brochure-USA11.pdf.
4. "Rocky Balboa Speech with Son Lyrics," http://www.justsomelyrics.com/2063678/Rocky-Balboa-speech-with-son-Lyrics.

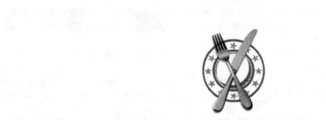